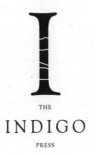

THE

INDIGO
PRESS

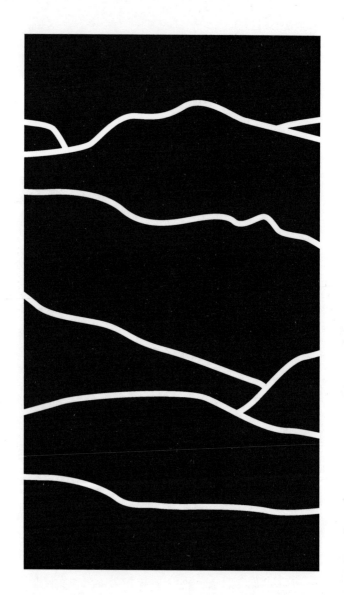

I CHOOSE ELENA

ON TRAUMA, MEMORY AND SURVIVAL

THE

INDIGO

PRESS

THE MOOD INDIGO
ESSAY SERIES

I CHOOSE ELENA

ON TRAUMA, MEMORY AND SURVIVAL

LUCIA OSBORNE-CROWLEY

THE

INDIGO

PRESS

MOOD INDIGO

An imprint of The Indigo Press

50 Albemarle Street

London W1S 4BD

www.theindigopress.com

The Indigo Press Limited Reg. No. 10995574

Registered Office: Wellesley House, Duke of Wellington Avenue

Royal Arsenal, London SE18 6SS

First published in Great Britain in 2019 by The Indigo Press

A CIP catalogue record for this book is available from the British Library

ISBN 978-1-9996833-9-9

eBook ISBN 978-1-911648-00-0

Design by www.salu.io

Typeset in Goudy Old Style by www.beyondwhitespace.com

Printed and bound in Great Britain

by TJ International, Padstow

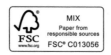

MIX
Paper from
responsible sources
FSC® C013056

To Elena, who taught me to love without suffering

CONTENTS

In order to rise
From its own ashes,
A phoenix
First
Must
Burn.

Octavia E. Butler

I

I buried the girl I had been because she ran into all kinds of trouble. I tried to erase every memory of her. But she is still there, somewhere.

Roxane Gay, *Hunger: A Memoir of (My) Body*

BEGINNINGS

Growing up, I was a gymnast. The serious kind. By the time I was ten, I had represented New South Wales at the national championships and won. At age twelve, I represented Australia at the world championships.

By fifteen, I was preparing for my second world championships. I trained relentlessly.

Every morning I drank raw eggs mixed with protein powder and milk. I was training so much that my body had started using my muscle mass for energy, which could result in my muscles atrophying. That's what the raw eggs were for: I needed to be consuming as much protein as possible to keep my muscles intact.

Weakness was the one thing we were all taught to avoid. I took this lesson seriously. No amount of eggs, protein bars, crunches, toe-points, handstand push-ups or weightlifts could deter me. I would push my body right to its limits, then further.

The kind of gymnastics I was doing required immense mental precision. I needed to synchronize wholly with my body, to pick up on every signal it sent me. I needed to master a very particular kind of mindfulness in order to step onto a velvet floor on a world stage, with five international judges ready to pick apart my every movement. My mind had to be so still that it could communicate with every pointed toe, every carefully balanced leg, every finger.

I had to be perfect, and it had to seem effortless. I had to be strong and powerful and graceful and light, all at the same time. I had to smile. To do all these things at once takes a kind of mind–body alignment that I have been dreaming of regaining ever since I stepped off the floor for the last time. My body and my mind, it seemed then, belonged wholly to me.

I was obsessed with this feeling. When I wasn't training, I took ballet classes to fill the time.

We called the gym our second home. For some of us, at times, it felt like a first home. Each year when we qualified for the national team, we would go on week-long training camps during which we would wake up at 5 a.m. to go for a long run, then do three training sessions throughout the day before crawling into sleeping bags placed atop crash mats on the gym floor. When we were slow to wake up, my coach would play Rihanna's 'Pon de Replay' on the gymnasium's enormous sound system.

I would be thrown in the air by another gymnast and do a double somersault and land perfectly. Sometimes the somersaults would be in the pike position, or the layout position, so you had to jump high and hard enough to rotate your stretched-out body twice before reaching the floor. Sometimes we did triple somersaults. Sometimes we did double layouts with a full twist in the first rotation.

We balanced our handstands on the hands of another gymnast and then morphed our bodies into overarch – a move in which you arch your back so much in the handstand that your feet touch your hands – while the gymnast holding us up slides into the splits. Sometimes we did the handstands with only one arm.

These manoeuvres are not just complicated but profoundly dangerous – gymnasts have died or been rendered paraplegic by a missed landing. We were all okay with danger; we were fearless. But the thing about staying safe as an athlete at that level is that your technique *must* be perfect. You need to know exactly how to jump; where your arms need to be at each point in a double somersault; how to hold your legs, your chest and your fingers so your handstand is unshakable.

I knew every inch of my body so well, could feel

every tiny sensation, could always tell if something was even just a little bit off.

Once I messed up a skill during training and I told my coach I hadn't slept well the night before; that I was nervous about a speech I had to give at school. His response was: If you are the athlete I know you can be, I should be able to wake you up in the middle of the night and you should be able to perform your skills, half asleep, with no warning.

I'm not sure if this was intended to be a metaphor; one he was using to teach me that at this level of the game, there is no excuse for mistakes. But I took it literally: I started waking myself up in the middle of the night and making sure I could hold a free handstand for three minutes straight.

The only time we got a day off was when a big competition was approaching. They call this 'tapering': a way of giving the body and the muscles a chance to recover from weeks and months of intense training so that all are in peak form for competition day. Sometimes these days were the hardest of them all; without training – the thing we spent the majority of our time doing – we had all these leftover hours to spend getting nervous about the competition.

During these tapering days, we were told to focus on mental preparation. We were taught by sports psychologists from the age of nine or ten how best to use the mental technique of 'visualization': a process in which we sit still, close our eyes and imagine ourselves – really imagine, including the sounds and smells and stomach flips – performing our routines.

During visualization, we would focus on the tricks or parts of the routine that frightened us the most, and we would make sure that we performed those elements flawlessly.

We were told to close our eyes and recall exactly what perfection felt like: the angle at which we left the floor, the feeling of the balls of our feet as we did our run-up, the sense once we were in the air of knowing that we had managed the jump and the rotation just so, the sense of knowing long before we hit the ground that we will land perfectly.

I learned so much about mindfulness, about muscle memory, about the wisdom of the body so early in my life, only to have it all taken from me, stored in some dark, dusty corner of my mind that I would not be brave enough to enter until a decade later.

Competition day would arrive. My Irish-British-Australian parents had bought a tiny gold four-leaf clover to sew into each of my competition leotards for good luck. I would wake up on the day of a competition and eat exactly what my coach had always instructed me: melted cheese on white rice. Carbs and protein, he would say. Nothing else.

We pulled on our competition leotards, sprayed our hair with bottles and bottles of hairspray to keep it in place, covered our faces in make-up to match our intricate leotards and our routines that told stories. On the warm-up floor, usually out the back end of an auditorium, I was always a mess of nerves. But then my coach would say, It's time, and we'd start the long walk down the corridor to the competition arena. During that walk, each and every time I did it the nerves would disappear.

During that walk I knew I could do what I needed to do. I knew I could do it perfectly. It's a feeling I have never been able to replicate.

We were always told to smile at the judges to get the best scores, told to smile even if we were hurting, even if we were exhausted. But for me, it was effortless. You couldn't stop me from beaming on that competition floor if you tried. I'm told that the top national judges called me *the smiling girl*.

During those years I never needed to manufacture my smile. I was one of the best athletes in my sport in the country and I knew it. But the thing about being a teenage girl is that at a certain point, the outside world intrudes on this narrative and it reconstructs your perception of your body without your knowledge or permission.

We wilt under the predatory gaze of men who turn us into objects for public consumption. We become so conspicuous in this light that we start to think it is all we are. In this light, we wish to be invisible.

In this light, we dream we will disappear.

I n Elena Ferrante's quartet, now known as the *Neapolitan* series, she tells the story of two young women, Elena and Lila, best friends and confidantes, growing up in Naples in the 1950s and 60s. The novels narrate the truth of a friendship: its love, its envy, its complexity, its nuance.

The story begins at the end, when Elena, the narrator, is in her sixties and Lila has gone missing. She receives this news as if it were a report of the morning weather. Because, she tells her reader, Lila always wanted to become invisible:

> It's been at least three decades since she told me she wanted to disappear without leaving a trace, and I'm the only one who knows what she means. She wanted to vanish; she wanted every one of her cells to disappear, nothing of her ever to be found.

Any person who has moved through the world with the body of a woman will know what it feels like to wish to be invisible. In the end, Lila never escapes this feeling. She finds a way to disappear.

I don't blame her. Overcoming this feeling is one of the hardest lessons a woman can learn. It is an ongoing act of survival.

What I am about to tell you is a story about

unlearning this desire to vanish: about insisting on inhabiting my body, about giving myself form and shape and substance. It is a story about learning how to be seen.

II

Why would anyone want to leave their body?
he laughed,
And in this moment, we had nothing in the world
in common.

Blythe Baird,
'For The Rapists
Who Called Themselves Feminists'

ENDINGS

It was August 2007, a rainy winter's night in Sydney. I was out on a Saturday night with three friends, at a dingy karaoke bar that smelled of must and damp and sweat.

We drank vodka cruisers and sang nasty songs about boys who were playing hard to get. I sang a truly awful rendition of Justin Timberlake's 'Cry Me a River' and, with no subtlety, tact or poetic integrity, inserted the name of the boy I was chasing into the end of every chorus. My friends joined in. It felt so good to find a space in which we could safely scream about the boys who had wronged us with no one we knew watching.

While gymnastics took up a great deal of my time, I had another life too. The life of a regular teenage girl. The life of a girl trying to figure out puberty and femininity and sex and alcohol and everything in between. When I wasn't training, I lived an exuberant double life as a high-achieving, extroverted high-school student surrounded by loving friends.

I played handball with the boys at recess to prove that I was *chill*. I was audacious and confident. One high-school friend tells me that the first time she met me, when we were eleven, I was lecturing my classmates about the differences between communism in theory and communism in practice.

I fell hard and fast for boys who had no interest in me and dedicated my time to signing in and out of MSN Messenger in the hope they would notice I was online. It never worked. Here's a hard-won lesson from my twenty-six-year-old self: if you have to remind someone that you exist, they are not worth your time.

In Year 8 I got my first boyfriend. He was in a band, liked all the same music I liked, and I was completely besotted. I can't remember if we ever really did anything together, but I do remember brimming with pride as I sat on his lap and held his hand at house parties in front of all our friends.

But then he was spotted kissing another girl on the bus. I was heartbroken. My dearest friend threw a basketball at his head.

I was elected vice-president of the student body, which, in my high school, was a big deal. I was hyperactive in the school community and spent time organizing Valentine's Day rose drives and school dances. I was thriving in every sense of the word. I studied hard. I made friends and I kept them. I would call their landlines from my landline every night after training, and we would talk for hours, even though we would see each other again the next morning. I scribbled Kelly Clarkson lyrics in my school diary during maths, while the boys in the class passed around notes rating the girls on a scale of one to ten for attractiveness and personality. Being a teenager is cut-throat.

The same year I was elected vice-president I befriended the boys in the year above me. I started going to their parties and standing outside nervously for twenty minutes before walking in, vodka cruisers in hand, ready to ingratiate myself with the in-crowd. One of these boys, of course, was the one I was singing about that night during 'Cry Me a River'.

At about 9 p.m. that night in 2007, we decided to leave the karaoke bar because we had run out of money. Emerging at the top of the creaky stairs, we found ourselves in the glow of Sydney's Pitt Street. In front of us stood the towering McDonald's on the corner. We were hungry. We crossed the road towards it.

A group of four grown men approached us and

started talking to us. Purposefully, I realized later, they distracted my three friends as a fifth, out of nowhere, appeared behind me and slipped his hand into mine. Come with me, he whispered.

The four other men closed in on my three friends and no one noticed us leave. He was gripping my hand so tightly I thought he might break my fingers. He marched me into McDonald's, towards a door on the left-hand side of the room. We went up one flight of stairs, where the public bathrooms were. He kept going.

He walked me up another flight of stairs to a dusty, disused bathroom. Perhaps it had once been for staff, or perhaps it was just an extra men's toilets the franchise no longer needed. It was empty, and deathly quiet.

He took me into a stall, locked the door and assaulted me, again, and again, and again. I had never had sex before so I had no reference point for any of what was happening to me apart from what I'd seen in movies, but I knew for certain that it was the sharpest and most severe pain I had ever experienced.

If you've read about trauma you will know that the human body's autonomic nervous system gives it three options in this kind of situation: fight, flight or freeze.

I lunged once at the latch of the stall door but he moved his body in front of it and didn't move from that position. Flight, my body instantly recognized, was not an option.

Fight. The man was about thirty-five, and made almost entirely of muscle. He looked like he had spent most of his twenties at the gym. I was still just a little over 40 kilos, true to my athletic dreams.

I tried once to push myself far enough away from him that I could reach around him for the door. At this point, he pulled out a Swiss army knife and held it against my throat. Fight was also out of the question.

When the first two options fail and the danger is still present, the autonomic nervous system sends a signal to the brain that death is imminent and the body begins to prepare itself.

The body releases its most powerful natural analgesic and cuts off signals from all major nerve endings.

The brain then enters a state of dissociation. In these moments, one feels distinctly as though one is floating above one's body, patiently watching, waiting, feeling nothing at all. The feeling of calm dissociation spreads from the mind to the muscles and veins themselves, right down to the bones.

Another element of the freeze response is referred to in trauma literature as 'collapse'. This also occurs the moment the body realizes that death has come for it. The collapse response involves all the muscles shutting down, becoming limp, no longer needed for escape because escape has been deemed impossible. The body stops fighting. It gives in. Once entirely loosened, the muscles will cease to resist whatever is trying to hurt the body and death will come faster. More mercifully.

The state of collapse is activated at the point of total helplessness. It is usually accompanied by a thought, or a sense, that the fight is over. I remember this moment clearly: as my attacker held the knife hard against my throat, I thought to myself: When he's finished, he's going to kill me.

In these calm moments the brain surveys the scenario one final time for possible escape routes. In most traumatic situations, it is this moment in which the body resigns itself to death that the mind finds a way to survive.

I noticed a glass bottle sitting to the right of the toilet bowl, leaning slightly against the door. I bent over – feeling, in that moment, none of the pain in my body – grabbed the bottle, and smashed it over the porcelain lid of the toilet bowl. This startled him for only a few seconds, but it was enough. As he tried to figure out the source of the loud smash, the flying glass and the reverberations as my elbow hit the door of the stall when it recoiled from the effort of breaking the glass, I reached for the door, unlocked it and ran away.

I ran down the stairs. I found my friends looking desperate, casting their eyes around the street wildly, panicked, wondering where I could have gone. Together, the four of us ran around the corner and I collapsed.

All I remember from those moments is the sound

of my gasping breath, the strength of my hands as I clutched my stomach, my pitchy sobs and the only words I could muster: It hurts.

My oldest friend sprung to her feet and ran in the direction of the attacker, but he was gone. None of us would ever see him again.

As she came back, a taxi pulled up with its yellow light on, and I remember insisting that I was fine and just needed to go home. I piled myself into the car and gave the driver my address, hoping against hope that on that particular night I had saved enough money from the karaoke bar for the ride home, like I usually did. My body shook uncontrollably in the back seat.

I snuck into the house, making sure my parents wouldn't notice me come in through the side entrance. I didn't want them to worry. My room was in the back of the house, with its own bathroom, so hiding from them was easy. I fell into the shower, bleeding everywhere, staring blankly into a tiled abyss and thinking only of the sound that thick glass makes when it smashes.

I got up the next morning as usual. I washed the stale cigarette smell out of my hair. I told my coaches I had twisted my ankle so I could stay away from the gym while the bruises healed. I went to school on the Monday and told stories about the cheesy pop songs we had sung about the embarrassing crushes we couldn't let go of. I waited for the bruises to fade and went back to training. I told no one. My friends knew that something had happened but I brushed off any questions they had and we never spoke about it again. I was too scared to revisit that night. We all were. We were just kids.

I was fifteen.

This was around the time my friends were losing their virginity to their high-school sweethearts and it was all we could talk about. I pushed the pain and the trauma of this event so far into the darkest corners of my mind that all I could think about those next few weeks was whether or not I was still a virgin.

What would I say the next time someone asked me? To say I'd never had sex would be a lie, but it was far preferable to recounting anything close to the truth. The truth was unspeakable.

I had been talking to a boy on Myspace who was older than me and had just graduated from my high school. I started going over to his house when his parents weren't home. After a few encounters, he asked me if I'd had sex before and I said no. I jumped at the opportunity.

That day I resolved the question of my virginity once and for all. It was 22 January 2008. I know this because it was the day Heath Ledger died, and we spoke about it in the car when he dropped me home.

That experience felt almost as bad as the rape itself, except there was even more shame because I had chosen it. My body burned for days and days afterwards, and I was left with a piercing pain in my abdomen.

Never again, I promised myself.

He drove me home and then stopped speaking to me, as many eighteen-year-old boys would do. I was crushed, probably in a desperately out-of-proportion way, because I thought that engaging in consensual sex would erase my assault. But it didn't work.

During that encounter the condom broke, so the next day I found myself, not yet sixteen, standing in a chemist waiting for the morning after pill. The pain in my abdomen was so severe that I fell to the ground as my friend and I left the chemist. So I went back to pretending nothing had happened, and promised myself I would never think or talk about sex again for as long as I lived. This strategy worked almost seamlessly for a while, but at my most vulnerable and volatile moments, parts of it would spill out of me. Once, I got drunk at a party and told an almost-complete stranger.

I was raped, I whispered to her, slurring. I didn't see her again until months later, when she showed up at a house party I was hosting, hugged me kindly and said, I'll never tell anyone. A friend and I got our drinks spiked when we were nineteen and I told her the story, over and over and over again, like I was a broken record stuck on a single graphic song.

When these pieces of the story leaked out of me, I barely recognized them as my own. I questioned whether the memory was real. I searched for it consciously but could find only fragments of it that refused to align themselves in a way that made sense to me. I convinced myself I had imagined it. This project made the random but semi-regular confessions to strangers all the more distressing. I was ashamed of admitting that this had happened to me, but then I would remind myself of the story I had created to numb the first shame: that it had never happened at all. I felt ashamed of a lie I hadn't told, but after a while I realized that the shame of thinking I had lied was easier to manage than the shame of admitting I hadn't.

Years later, I would come across *The Body Keeps the Score*, by Dr Bessel van der Kolk. The culmination of a life's work, the book gives a neurobiological, psychosocial and psychiatric account of post-traumatic stress. It outlines the ways in which traumatic events have lasting impacts on the immune system, the nervous system, the muscular system and the brain.

About two years after my assault, I was struck down by unbearable abdominal pain. I vomited from the force of it. I started to bleed everywhere. Blood poured down my legs and pooled around my feet. I passed out. I began to have a constant, intrusive thought about a knife being plunged into my vagina. This is what trauma scholars call a 'felt memory'; it is my body's way of recalling how the rape felt, but because the memory itself is locked away, the brain comes up with an alternative memory to represent the feeling. As far as I know, my attacker did not actually plunge his knife into me, but this is how my body interpreted the feeling that my mind refused to acknowledge.

This happens just before the actual fragments of the memory return to the conscious mind. It is a sign that the memory is catching up with you. Hunting you down. I kept running, I ran faster, from him, from the memory, from the pain. But it didn't work. I started having nightmares about the attack, in tiny fragments, and would wake up screaming and shaking, and ashamed that I had let him back into my head.

Over the next few years my body started to break down, physically, in a way that I assumed to be entirely unconnected to the event I had tried so hard to forget. I lost my sense of balance and any degree of connection to my body. I stopped being able to perform gymnastics routines I had long ago perfected. My coaches and fellow athletes knew something was wrong, but when they asked I couldn't explain it. I lost all sense of my physical self. I started injuring myself at training as a consequence of being unable to know precisely where the different parts of me begun and ended. I remember picking myself up after disastrously under-rotating on a round-off-flip layout and casting my eyes around the gym in search of something that could explain the fall. Had the mats shifted underneath me? Had I tripped on another athlete's abandoned ankle strap? No answers presented themselves.

In trauma discourse, this is described as a loss of

'proprioception': the ability of the mind to gauge effectively the relationship between the body and everything external to it. Proprioception is how the mind tells the body how to move through the world, how to control its most delicate movements, how much space it takes up.

I read once that the reason cats can shape-shift to fit themselves into remarkably small spaces is that the tips of their whiskers are biologically coded to be exactly the same width as the widest parts of their body. They use them as a kind of proprioceptive radar. All of a sudden I was without that sense, unable to orient myself, never quite sure which parts of the world I could fit into and which I couldn't. I had a major fall in the try-outs for my second world championships. I injured my ankle so badly that my sports doctor told me I would be lucky if I went for a jog again. I have barely set foot on a gym floor since.

I have also learned from reading the psychiatrist Peter Levine that something else important happened in my brain on the night of the attack. The ways in which we store memories can be broadly classified into two categories: declarative memories and procedural memories. Declarative memories are the ones we can explicitly recall, fully formed. They have been stored in the brain as narrative experiences, as stories about our lives. Procedural memories, on the other hand, are subconscious. They live in the body, in the muscles and joints and blood. The body remembers how to conduct certain procedures without having to think about them. This is 'muscle memory'.

So there I was, fifteen years old, with ten years' worth of procedural memories in my back pocket. My muscles knew the feeling of a perfect handstand, of the correct take-off for a somersault. I never had to think about these things, the instructions lived deep inside my bones.

But what happened on that night in the bathroom in 2007 was so acutely life-threatening that it engendered in my brain a new, much more powerful form of procedural memory: the knowledge of how the body freezes when it needs to escape, the hyper-vigilance with which the body senses danger, the desperate need to run away. Because these procedural memories are, from an evolutionary perspective, much more important than everyday tasks such as showering, getting dressed, making a cup of tea, they take over. The psychiatrist Robert Jay Lifton describes these new, overriding procedural memories as an 'indelible image'. A 'death imprint'.

Entering the state of collapse is useful in moments of real danger, but once we live through it once and survive, the brain can rewire itself to be on high-alert in any subsequent moments of helplessness, no matter how serious or life-threatening they are, and collapse can become a state we enter regularly. We find ourselves re-entering a frozen state at the passing of a loud car, a door slammed too heavily, a sudden burst of laughter from a nearby table at a restaurant.

My body's fight, flight or freeze response became my only form of procedural memory; like trauma itself, it destroys everything in its path. Muscle memories of perfect technique and form that I had spent my entire life building were erased in seconds by the need to survive.

The loss of my athletic self was a profound one, and for months I pretended I could get past it, return to my gymnastics world as if nothing had happened. Deep down I knew it was over, but accepting this was devastating.

I am like this with most things. Acceptance and loss are profoundly difficult for me to process. I am overly sentimental. I hoard things. I cling to memories even when they have become so distant they feel like fantasies. I cling to fantasies as though they are memories. As David Foster Wallace famously wrote, 'Everything I've ever let go of has claw marks on it.' Sometimes I think that should be written on my tombstone.

As I was processing the fact that my athletic career was over, I began experiencing a series of organic failures that grew, developed and shape-shifted over the seven years that followed. First my bladder, then my appendix, then my uterus, then my bowel. My body, which had once been so obedient, started to unravel.

I watched this happen as if I were standing outside myself, as if I were watching a broken-down car splutter to a halt and burst into flames. I had no means whatsoever of understanding what was happening, so instead of inspecting the damage, I ran from it, left the shell of my body where it had fallen and ignored it for years.

Here's what I now know my body was doing while I pretended I could wish it away. When an everyday event concludes, the brain places it in a sequence, understanding how each moment, each event, led to the next, and analysing the experience based on this narrative.

But traumatic memories get stuck. They cannot be rearranged into logical narratives, and instead remain trapped in the brain as flashes of light, sound and smell – rogue fragments of an unbearable memory that leak out at the mind's weakest moments. As a result, instead of understanding these stimuli as past events, the brain reacts to these fragments of memory as though the event is still happening. The part of the brain responsible for separating the past from the present – the hippocampus – becomes dysfunctional and the brain re-enters fight, flight or freeze every time it is reminded of the experience. The past bleeds into the present, again and again and again.

The hippocampus is closely connected to the amygdala, the part of the brain responsible for our most basic emotions: fear, joy, safety, grief. If the hippocampus fails to store away a memory as a past experience, it forces us to relive the memory every time the amygdala senses danger – whether that be a sense of actual danger or a fragment of the traumatic memory itself, which can be as benign as a certain song, a particular bird call, the smash of a wine glass knocked over at a dinner party.

Unlike other memories that can be safely stored away by the hippocampus, traumatic memories stay alive. They lie in wait and then move through us like breath. A death imprint.

This confusion then extends to the entire nervous system. The body's autonomic nervous system has two separate modes: the sympathetic nervous system and the parasympathetic nervous system. The sympathetic nervous system is the fight-or-flight response, and the parasympathetic nervous system its opposite: its job is to calm the body down when the threat has passed.

When a person is traumatized, their sympathetic nervous system becomes disastrously overactive. It kicks into fight, flight or freeze at the smallest hint of danger or reminder of a traumatic event. The parasympathetic nervous system becomes weak and dysfunctional: its usual tricks for calming the body down degrade over time as the sympathetic nervous system takes over.

This has a profoundly damaging effect on the body when it is allowed to continue for weeks, months or years. The autonomic nervous system suspends all physical functions not considered necessary for escape, and sends blood and oxygen to the major muscle groups, ready to run. Anything not needed for immediate escape is brought to a standstill.

This means that in traumatized people, the body's primary organs - the stomach, the liver, the kidneys, the bowel - freeze up, sometimes for hours at a time, sometimes every day, whenever the autonomic nervous system is triggered by a memory or a flash of fear. These organs then have to restart once the parasympathetic nervous system kicks in. This leads to an exhausting process of near-constant stagnation and rebirth. Eventually, the systems and organs start to wither under the weight of it.

The longer a physical assault or accident is held in the nervous system, the muscles and the brain, without being addressed or treated, the more likely it is that it will manifest as a systemic physical disorder or dysfunction. The patient faces a future defined by illness as penance for being unable to escape an unbearable past.

Medical professionals now believe that the digestive system's dysfunctional response to untreated trauma can be one of the causes of abdominal disorders such as irritable bowel syndrome, Crohn's disease and endometriosis. New research suggests that it is possible that the long-term physiological impacts of trauma can also cause multiple sclerosis, migraines, fibromyalgia, some cancers and generalized chronic pain.

This research is in its early stages and, of course, there are other causes for these conditions. But for the first time, the medical profession is acknowledging that untreated trauma can lead to one – or more – of these disabilities.

It had never occurred to me that my physical ailments, all appearing in the same part of me, at the same time, could have a common cause.

And perhaps they don't. There is no exact formula for causation, no matter how desperately we might wish for one. My chronic physical illnesses could have been caused by any number of things, or an intricate combination of several factors, or just bad luck. I'll never know for sure.

But there is one thing I finally know to be true: one way or another, the body keeps the score.

III

This home is empty now. –

Rupi Kaur, 'I'm taking my body back'

ABSTRACTIONS

In December 2009, two years after the assault, I was hospitalized for acute abdominal pain associated with an alarming amount of bleeding and vomiting. A sexual assault specialist would tell me nearly a decade later that this timing is precisely what she would expect to see in the development of physiological symptoms of sexual trauma.

Years later, I would be diagnosed with endometriosis and Crohn's disease, both of which are organic disorders that doctors believe might be connected to untreated trauma. But the process of getting to these diagnoses was disheartening and torturous and humiliating. I remember so clearly the day it all began: 17 November 2009; I sat in a Sydney emergency department coiled over myself in pain, wondering what on earth could have happened to me. I didn't realize, then, how many more times I would have to do this.

The doctors were confused. My symptoms didn't add up neatly. They couldn't explain the vomiting. My urine sample showed an abnormally high white blood cell count and I had a fever but it didn't seem like an infection. I saw three different doctors that night, each with a furrowed brow and a barely veiled air of impatience. I felt frightened that they didn't know what was wrong with me. I felt exhausted from the fear and morphine. I felt guilty that I was making the doctors work so hard.

By the early hours of that morning, unable to find a more suitable explanation, the doctors had decided to treat me for a urinary tract infection. They filled my body with intravenous antibiotics; the sound of the drip mesmerized my addled mind.

But the pain didn't go away. It would take many more emergency room admissions before I was referred to a specialist. Each time, I would sit for hours on the green chairs of the waiting room, in between being carted to ultrasounds and doctors' rooms and blood tests. They would each present something slightly worrying – inflammation in my blood, strange movements on my ultrasound – but nothing conclusive. So they would treat me, again, for a UTI or a pelvic infection and send me on my way. I got the sense that they were glad to see the back of me.

On one of those nights in the emergency room, the pain was so severe that I could barely breathe or speak. I briefly lost consciousness on the sticky green chairs. The doctors thought I might have appendicitis. I didn't.

After this admission, I was encouraged to see a gynaecological specialist. I complied. I made an appointment with a woman whose name escapes me now, and whose face I can barely remember. In fact, I remember almost nothing about that appointment except the alarm in the woman's voice when I explained my symptoms to her. I told her I was in pain almost all the time. I estimated it was about an eight out of ten. I explained that no, it didn't come in waves. It was constant. I learned the word 'collicky'.

I told her it was very sharp for most of the day, like daggers. I told her that it sometimes dulled and felt more like period pain or the muscular pain I remembered from my gymnast days. In those moments, I said, it was probably only a six out of ten.

She looked worried. As the conversation wore on, my guilt expanded and I started to amend my experience to relieve the pressure I imagined she felt. I didn't tell her about how frequently the pain induced vomiting. I didn't tell her about the bleeding. Or the nausea. Still, she was alarmed. She said I needed a laparoscopy to find out what was going on. I told her I was too busy. She said it was urgent. She handed me a letter addressed to the triage department of the ER, instructing them to admit me immediately and prepare me for surgery. I told her I didn't want to. She told me I could be in real danger.

The surgery found nothing. They checked for ovarian cysts, but I had none. They checked my appendix again, but it was fine. The gynaecological surgeon was impatient with me. I see so many young women who overstate their symptoms and won't accept it when they find they are perfectly healthy, he said. It felt unjust. I wanted to protest, I wanted to tell him that I had tried to avoid being here at all, that I had said I was too busy. I did not choose this, I wanted to tell him, again and again and again. I would not choose this for anyone.

But my body was full of anaesthetic; the nausea from it so strong I was sure I would vomit if I opened my mouth. I wanted to stand up for myself, but I was too sick. Too tired. I fell asleep, feeling angry and confused, and dreamed about being eaten by human-sized cockroaches.

I lived like this for months. I was in and out of hospital every few weeks for the rest of that year. My existence was divided into the days and nights I spent in hospital beds and the weeks I spent clinging desperately to the functional, high-speed life I had perfected in the years before. I kept trying to go to lectures, to speak up in tutorials, to hold down my call-centre job. I pretended I wasn't sick, with pain and desperation bubbling awfully close to the surface but never breaking through.

After some months of this, the facade of competence started to fracture. My sadness turned into anxiety and I stopped going out. The pain got worse; sometimes it was so bad I couldn't move my legs. My iron stores plummeted from the bleeding. I lost my appetite. I barely ever made it to class. From what I can recall of those months, I think I mostly just lay on my couch with a hot-water bottle for each side of my abdomen and watched *Titanic* on repeat, crying like clockwork when Rose says, I'd rather be his whore than your wife.

I remember oscillating between total resignation and total panic, one moment feeling exhausted and cynical and the next, thoroughly convinced I was dying. Cutting through all of my madness was pure confusion, constantly wondering how it could be that my body was being assailed by a malevolent predator that no one could name.

I had more surgeries – endoscopies, colonoscopies, cystoscopies, a few more laparoscopies. They suggested irritable bowel syndrome. They checked my appendix a third time. 'Due diligence.'

I had more tests, too – ultrasounds, MRIs, pap smears, blood tests, urine tests, STD screens, X-rays, HIV tests. I had my first internal ultrasound when

I was nineteen. When the young male doctor explained how it would work, and the fear of penetration danced across my face, he paused, and then said softly, I have never understood why young women feel so uncomfortable about these ultrasounds but are happy to have sex with multiple men in their spare time.

My understanding of the complexities of gender politics was puerile. But I felt the sting of it somewhere very deep inside me, somewhere my conscious thoughts could barely reach.

As 2010 wore on the saga continued. I saw so many specialists and doctors and surgeons that I stopped trying to remember their names or their faces. I perfected my story. I learned that each pause I allowed between question and answer made me an increasingly untrustworthy witness. I learned the true meaning of statements like 'That all sounds very strange' and 'I'm surprised you manage to make it to work if the pain is that bad' and 'Why don't you calm down and start from the beginning'.

I learned to detect each tiny morsel of the phrase *I don't believe you*, no matter how veiled by sympathetic smiles or how fragmented by furious note-taking. I adopted a professionalism they lacked; my answers became clinical and unfeeling, my descriptions matter-of-fact.

I handed out my histories to stranger after stranger until I barely recognized them – my medical history, my family history, my academic record, my employment status, my mental health history, my sexual proclivities. I was not yet whole enough to deflect the doctors' disapproval. Instead, I internalized it.

I felt ashamed of myself for needing help. I felt ashamed of my imaginary pain. Sometimes, I would sit in appointments and convince myself that perhaps I really was imagining it. But then, a few hours later, the pain would come back and I would take myself to a bathroom and find myself bleeding heavily through my underwear, down my legs, into my socks, until I could feel it beneath my feet. I would sit on the tiled floor and wonder what to do, would watch the blood pool beneath me and wonder how I could ever leave the stall.

I would be lying if I said that these moments didn't sometimes spark intrusive thoughts about another thing I wasn't sure if I had imagined. There were times when I sat there, wishing I could disappear, and I thought to myself: I have only seen this much blood once before. But as soon as I regained control over my thoughts, I mopped up the memory, got myself clean and kept going.

Again and again, doctors asked me if I was feeling stressed, or anxious, or depressed, or panicked. I realize now that they were suggesting these things were the cause of my pain, but at the time the question felt insultingly obvious. Of course I feel stressed, I wanted to yell at them, my body is tearing itself apart and no one can tell me why.

After months of this, I remember sitting in an indistinguishable specialist's office and being told I needed to go to a 'pain clinic'. The woman explained to me gently that sometimes, when a person has been in pain for a long time, their mind loses its ability to craft 'appropriate' pain responses, firing thousands of pain signals when it only needs one, turning a stubbed toe into a day's agony. I clearly remember not understanding a word of this, but it felt legitimizing. It also felt hopeful; I was promised expert psychologists who could train my mind so completely that I would no longer experience pain. To a girl desperate to get back to herself, it sounded terrific.

The pain clinic was all white walls, sterile smells and bearded male psychiatrists. In my first appointment, I started the story I had rehearsed. My symptoms, my history, my surgeries. One psychiatrist explained that 'young women' were often referred to pain clinics when doctors decided their conditions were 'psychosomatic'. I had never heard that word before but I got his message loud and clear: I had spent months trying to convince doctor after doctor that I was losing my body, and they all thought I was losing my mind.

At nineteen, realizing that everyone around me thought my problem was psychological was the hardest part of all. Another psychiatrist at the clinic explained to me that some mental conditions are so powerful that they can begin to control the body, to manifest themselves in increasingly physical ways. I did not doubt that it was true, but I didn't believe it was true for me. My problem was not that I could use my mind to control my body. It was that for the first time in my life, I couldn't.

I persevered with the pain clinic for a few months before making an excuse to cancel an appointment and avoiding their calls for a year. I'm sure it would have been very helpful, had I been ready for it. But I wasn't, and so I kept running.

After I abandoned the clinic, my symptoms got worse. I started having acute episodes more frequently. I could never predict when they would come on. Once I was on an evening walking tour while on holiday with my sister, standing in a graveyard near a church, a young guide telling us a story about a ghost dog of some description – my memory fails me at this point – and I started to feel light-headed. The pain in my abdomen came on like lightning, my muscles contracted, my legs felt wobbly. I rushed off to a bathroom in a nearby pub, barely making it down the stairs, and locked myself in a cubicle. I lost my vision, and then my consciousness.

Years later, a surgeon friend of mine would tell me that many doctors don't take female pain particularly seriously. At the time, I wasn't sure if I believed him. Could that be true? Do people really think like that?

But now I know that the truth is this: studies have consistently found that doctors working in emergency rooms take women less seriously than men. Women who present to an emergency department with acute pain are less likely to be given effective painkillers than men reporting the same amount of pain. Even when women are prescribed pain relief by emergency doctors, they wait longer to receive it.

A study by Swedish academic Ann-Sophie Backman at the Karolinska University Hospital's Clinical Epidemiology Unit showed that a woman presenting to an emergency department was less likely to have her condition classified as 'urgent'. She was also more likely to spend significantly longer waiting in emergency wards than men who arrived at the same time with similar complaints.

A study by Diane E Hoffman and Anita Tarzian published in the *Journal of Law, Medicine and Ethics* showed that doctors are more likely to dismiss complaints of acute pain when they come from women. Another study from Healthline showed that when female pain is recognized and treated, it is treated less aggressively than the same degree of pain reported by men.

A UK study by John Guillebaud, professor of reproductive health at University College London, found that women presenting to emergency with pain will wait an average of sixteen minutes longer than men presenting with the same degree of pain. Women are also given smaller doses of pain relief than men who report the same degree of discomfort. Research cited by Hoffman and Tarzian has found that doctors are more likely to assume that female pain is a result of 'emotional causes', whereas male pain is presumed to be a result of a physical problem.

When doctors do consider that a woman's ailment may be a physical one, she is often presumed to be suffering from a gynaecological problem, which is less likely to be treated with pain relief, according to a study by Esther Chen, an emergency medicine doctor at Zuckerburg San Francisco General Hospital. I'd be willing to bet there's also an element of the profoundly inaccurate but deeply held belief that women should be blamed for any irregularities in their sexual health.

But far too often doctors never get past the point of presuming there is a psychological problem with the woman before them. So doctors refer her to a counsellor and send her home, still in pain, still potentially in danger, still completely unaware of what is wrong with her, and having just been told she's imagining things again.

I hear so many stories about being that woman. I have been that woman, again and again and again: riding home from hospital in a taxi, in pain I physically cannot bear without yelling, legs shaking, unable to move, having just been told that there is absolutely nothing wrong with me.

How could that be?

There is also a widely held belief that women are more likely to go to the doctor with less serious complaints than men, and therefore, when they do go to the doctor, they are taken less seriously. But a 2011 report from the Institute of Medicine shows that women and men are equally likely to consult doctors for conditions relating to pain; we also now know, contrary to cultural belief, that women actually have a higher pain tolerance than men. This evidence runs counter to deep-seated assumptions about the fragility and sensitivity of women – studies show that their pain is more likely to be seen as 'hysterical' or 'exaggerated' – and from our corresponding assumptions about the stoicism of men. Each of these studies bears out, to a frightening degree, the experience I had with doctors over the ten years in which I was hunting for a solution to my suffering.

Once I learned of these patterns, I filled out an elaborate legal document that allows a patient to access all of their hospital records. I collected the thick pile of medical records with bees in my throat. I cringed as I looked at how many hospital admissions they represented, how many hours of waiting in emergency rooms for nothing and no one, the indignity of it all.

As I leafed through the pages and pages of records, I saw just how naive I had been. Doctors' notes included comments like 'some guarding in response to pain but seems voluntary'; 'patient seems well enough; nothing organically wrong'.

Those scribbled notes haunt me in my sleep like a ghost, representing every experience of being disbelieved, right there on the page, in black and white.

The notes ended with comments such as 'Lucia's pain and discomfort was successfully managed and she is well and stable.' My pain and discomfort had not been successfully managed. I was not well and stable. I was a disaster.

The notes speak repeatedly about my sex life, about the possibility of sexually transmitted diseases. I kept insisting I didn't have any, that this wasn't possible. There are several separate reports of the pathologies that later came back regarding those supposed infections. I turn the pages over and over and each one said the same thing:

Negative.

Negative.

Negative.

Negative.

Negative.

And I turned the final page. Negative.

On not a single one of those occasions did I have a sexually transmitted infection. That's several courses of intravenous antibiotics I was given because doctors associate female abdominal pain with promiscuity.

It is important at this juncture to make one thing clear. That my pain was not taken seriously is certainly how I experienced these years of medical treatment. But I am also a journalist, and facts matter a great deal to me. While writing this book, I have spoken to doctors who have told me that if you present to emergency with abdominal pain as a woman, medics will immediately turn their attention to gynaecological emergencies first because they can be fatal much more quickly than other conditions. So doctors will immediately check for ectopic pregnancies and other gynaecological conditions that are life-threatening and require urgent surgical intervention.

So now I understand why doctors often jumped to conclusions about my sexual health. But it doesn't explain why, when those conclusions turned out to be wrong, they gave up on me altogether.

Once, I was sitting in a specialist's office and she said, Wow, it really doesn't take a lot for the wheels to fall off your cart; have you considered a psych analysis?

I wanted to defend myself but I knew if I made a sound, the tears in my throat would well up and reach my eyes and prove the very thing she was accusing me of: being weak, indulgent, playing victim.

At one point in the medical notes, a doctor wrote: 'The laparoscopy was normal and photos of the internal organs were given to Lucia to show her the organs are fine.' It turned out that my endometriosis specialist, when he later examined those photos, could see evidence of the disease. The doctor reported in a separate letter about that visit: '[Lucia] was thoroughly investigated including a diagnostic laparoscopy which was noted to be entirely normal.'

Next I leafed through the stack of blood results that had come in the package of hospital records. Every single time I went through emergency the doctors told me that all my blood work had come back 'relatively normal', so there was nothing to investigate there. This is only a half-truth.

In every single one of the fifteen blood results I have records of, bar one, my lymphocyte levels were abnormally high. In many, my eosinophils were also abnormally high. In some, my neutrophil levels were abnormally high too. In some, my white-blood-cell count was higher than it should have been. Each of these indicators tells us about how the white blood cells in the body are behaving. Each of them is raised when the body is going through an inflammatory process. Both endometriosis and Crohn's diseases are inflammatory conditions.

I'm also struck by the number of times my notes reflect that I reported the pain and vomiting became worse during my period. That, along with the telltale signs of an inflammatory disease in my blood work, should have pointed the doctors to endometriosis. At the end of the stack of papers, I found a number of ultrasound reports of my abdomen, all of which were reported to be 'normal'. However, the ultrasound reports themselves – which I now have access to – consistently showed a large amount of free fluid in my Pouch of Douglas, which often indicates there is endometriosis in that area.

In another act of determination to prove that my illness was brought on by my audacity to be having sex at eighteen, when I reported an episode of bleeding so extreme that I passed out, the doctors decided I had had a miscarriage. This was unlikely, I explained, as I had a long-term partner and was very responsible with the contraceptive pill, but that didn't seem to matter all that much to them.

It seems so cruel to sit in front of a stack of old scribbled notes and blood tests and pathology results that tell you that you weren't, as the doctors said, 'in fact completely healthy', but that you had a serious and permanent condition and desperately needed treatment.

I cried for how much they had taken from me – my autonomy, my health, my resilience – and I couldn't decide whether to put the medical records away somewhere safe or burn them so no one would ever know how much they degraded me, how foolish I had been.

The problem was not medicine itself; the answer was right there on the pages. The problem was that no one was looking for it.

A few days before Christmas in 2010, I lay in a hospital bed after another emergency room visit and another surgical procedure. I felt exhausted. A psychiatric nurse kept coming in and out of my room, asking me about my plans for the holidays. A gynaecological surgeon came to my bedside and told me he thought he knew what was wrong with me.

He explained that he thought I had a gynaecological condition that had affected my uterus, my ovaries, my bladder, and possibly other organs too. It was called endometriosis, he said. Even after months of exploration into every crevice of my body and my personal history, I had never even heard the word before. I didn't understand what he was saying, but he seemed so sure of it. I felt comfortable in his presence.

He explained that endometriosis is a disease of the tissue in the uterus. In women who have the condition, the tissue grows outside the uterus, in all sorts of unsuitable places. The tissue – called endometrial cells – can grow on various abdominal organs: the bladder, the bowel, the ovaries, the kidneys.

The abnormal cells spread, and can grow so much that they overrun these organs like a cancerous carpet.

If it is particularly aggressive, the tissue can reach such a critical mass that it stops the organs from moving around in the body, trapping them and suffocating them until they can barely function. I wouldn't learn this until years later, speaking to a doctor after an internal ultrasound – which I was very accustomed to by that stage – who told me my endometriosis was so bad that it had brought my whole abdominal infrastructure to a standstill.

The endometriosis, my surgeon explained, could be so damaging that it can cause other organic problems too. Kidneys, bladder, bowels. The endometriosis will destroy their functionality as it grows and spreads. And, he told me, it can be very painful.

He did the surgery and found a great deal of endometriosis as well as a related inflammatory bladder condition.

Sitting in his cosy surgical office, he showed me images of my organs from the surgery. It looked like an abandoned battleground: everything torn apart, shredded, bloody. Broken.

He paused and let me process the images. He watched my face as it moved from shock, to fear, to relief.

You didn't make this up, he said. I'm not surprised you've been in so much pain.

In *The Empathy Exams*, Leslie Jamison reflects on what we mean when we talk about empathy. Is it enough to simply imagine the pain of others? Is it enough to imagine what you would feel like to exist in their body, in their life? Or is it more than that: is it the ability to not only imagine a person's pain but to then calculate exactly what that person needs from you in order to alleviate a small piece of it? Reading this, all I could think about was that appointment. Even though I had never once communicated to that doctor, never even hinted, that my biggest fear was not being believed, he knew. And not only did he know, but he knew that he needed to legitimize my pain by voicing it. He knew my fears about my credibility ran so deep that he needed to wait until he had proof, hard evidence, of my disease before he could reassure me.

He never uttered the words until he knew they would mean something. He needed to puncture a self-doubt that was more pervasive even than I recognized.

I needed people . . . to deliver my feelings back to me in a form that was legible. Which is a superlative kind of empathy to seek, or to supply: an empathy that rearticulates more clearly what it's shown.

That is how Jamison described her expectations of empathy. That is exactly how I felt about that conversation with my surgeon; that he was delivering something to me that I was too vulnerable even to know I needed.

He explained to me that my condition was aggressive,

and that we needed a treatment plan. That it might affect my fertility, and certainly my quality of life. He explained that there was no cure, that there was barely even a consensus on a cause. He said I was very unlucky.

He told me he was sorry.

He told me we needed to do another surgery to scrape out the diseased tissue. He said it was likely the cells had torn holes in the linings of my organs; that I probably had masses of scar tissue floating around inside my body like castaway lifeboats. He explained that the surgery would be hard, but that it would help.

I loathed the thought of another surgery but I revelled in his certainty. He had answers. He had a plan. I waited, and I think I even started to feel better.

He explained that he would also inject Botox into my bladder to stop it from attacking itself and to ease the pain. He explained that Botox was a good tool to create an artificial barrier in the battleground my abdominal organs had become. I trusted him.

It was mid-2012. The surgery was scheduled for the week following our appointment. The pain was becoming unbearable, and I ached for respite. I was almost excited.

When I came out of surgery, the doctors told me it had been worse than they thought. I was re-anaesthetized to keep me under for the several hours they needed to rid my body of the disease. I vomited for two hours after I woke up. I was so tired.

The surgeons explained that the disease had created lesions and tears all throughout my abdomen, and that it had taken them hours to patch me up. They told me my bladder was angry and sore. They told me my appendix was covered in endometriosis, so they decided it would be easier to just remove it rather than spend hours scraping the diseased tissue from its walls. Finding this out caused me to feel a funny sort of grief: I longed for the return of an organ I had never needed, never used, one which was imbued with value only when its removal became a physical manifestation of my profound loss of control.

The next morning the doctors removed the catheter from my body and began the testing they were required to do before letting me go home. It was just some routine checks, the nurses explained. They had to make sure that my bladder was working and that all my critical organs were functional. Unfortunately, my bladder was so damaged from the surgery and the anaesthetic that it didn't work. I failed all the tests. It was too dangerous to send me home. I stayed in hospital for days, hoping each morning there would be my last. After a week of this, my surgeon sent me home with my catheter and some complicated testing devices.

You've been in hospital too long, he explained. You'll only get sicker.

He told me to go home and rest for a week, and come back, and they would disconnect the wires and see if my body was ready to work again. He told me he wasn't surprised. Your organs have been through so much, he said. They are exhausted. They've got no fight left in them.

I went home and lay in the spare room of my parents' house for a week and cried. I wasn't allowed any codeine in case it damaged my organs further, so I soaked in the bath for hours at a time, the steaming hot water my only hope for a natural painkiller. I barely moved. My sister was in the final throes of her thesis, but she set up a temporary working space in my parents' living room to keep me company. At regular intervals she walked to the local shops to buy me cranberry juice: the one thing I was allowed to use to fight off developing infection.

I had panic attack after panic attack, convinced my organs had abandoned me for good. I called the nurses daily and implored them to help me. I cried often. I craved distraction. I begged for relief. I needed my body back. One night I called a friend in tears and told him I didn't know if I could stand any more pain. I am ashamed to admit this, but in that moment I really meant it. I didn't know how to keep going. What if I don't get through this? I asked.

I'm not sure what I was asking exactly. My condition wasn't severe enough to be life-threatening, but I felt as though it had the potential to change me in some deep, irreversible way.

You will, he said.

How do you know?

I was so used to people telling me it would be okay, that I would recover, that I could return to my life as a 20-year-old as if nothing had happened. I braced myself for one of those soliloquies.

He sighed heavily.

Because you don't have a choice.

It was the first time I felt as though someone understood how far away I was.

This went on for weeks. My parents looked after me tirelessly and constantly found new ways to distract me. This was a routine they would perfect over the years that followed. Every day they brought me things to read that they knew reminded me of my other life: the newspaper, the *Economist*, novels I loved. In fact, years later I would be lying in a sterile hospital bed, unable to move or walk, and my parents would bring me the first of Ferrante's *Neapolitan* novels. It's only thanks to them that I got to choose Elena.

When I went back into hospital, they disconnected my body from its helpers and it came to life again. It was August 2012 and the winter sun felt as though it was shining only for me. My sister took me to Nando's and I ate solid food for the first time in two weeks. We laughed for hours, filled with relief, and then I slept for three days straight.

I have had four more surgeries since that one, each

an attempt to rid my body of its disease faster than it can grow. Each with a doctor I trust. Each one has been successful, but the condition is unstoppable. My doctor says that soon we will have to start talking about freezing my eggs; it is unlikely they will survive many more years in the war zone my body has become.

In 2014, I found myself pregnant. I was on the contraceptive pill and I was strict with myself about taking it at the same time every day, but like everyone else, I am human. I don't know for sure how this pregnancy happened. It's possible that I missed a pill, or took one too late. My doctors were astounded, delighted that I had been able to conceive despite my rampant disease. They told me seriously to consider keeping the baby because I might never get pregnant again. I was twenty-two.

But this is a miracle, they said, again and again and again.

Why would a doctor encourage a sick person, a girl who struggles every single day to look after herself, to bring a new person into the world? And why did this male doctor think he had any right to counsel me on my decision as to whether or not I should have a child at twenty-two? He had never even asked if I wanted children at all. Why would he presume to be a part of a decision like that?

One doctor also told me that sometimes when

women get pregnant for the first time, the disease slows down. Sometimes it goes away entirely.

I held firm eye contact with him and said, No, a baby is not a Band-Aid.

I was so young and my then-partner and I were living in my parents' house and I had been in and out of hospital for five years and my life felt like a mess so I got the abortion anyway.

I am an anxious person and that day in 2014, as soon as I realized my period was late, I ran home and took a pregnancy test. I went to the doctor first thing the next morning and he told me it was extremely early in the pregnancy. The abortion clinic wouldn't let me have the operation until I was six weeks' pregnant. I hung up the phone in the tiny office of the local paper I worked for and stared at a notepad I had been scribbling headline ideas on the day before. I wondered how I would get through those next two weeks, knowing there was something miraculous happening inside me, something I had never wanted but had morphed into a fantasy after being told I couldn't have it, wondering if I might look back on this time and think how lucky I was, wondering if I could ever forgive myself for what I was about to do, wondering if I had the strength to do it at all.

Eventually, the weeks passed and I woke up on the morning of my appointment. I woke up scared and heavy with guilt. I dragged myself to the clinic. I thought about the fact that after all these years of emergency surgery, I was having one that was planned. One that I had chosen. How did I end up here?

I am strongly pro-choice and resisted any shame the doctors or nurses associated with this decision. I managed not to hate myself as the male protestors outside the clinic lunged at me as I walked in. But I did truly despise myself later that day, when I got home, with stomach cramps that left me curled in the foetal position in the shower, bleeding, admonishing myself for making a choice that caused extra pain when I had so much already.

And also, in the smallest, most apolitical part of me, believing what the doctors had said, asking myself: Why had I given up an opportunity that might never come around again?

I wish I could say this experience didn't hurt me, but it did.

The surgery cost me hundreds of dollars. I told almost no one. So it went: more surgery. More trauma. More pain. More secrets.

I was deeply disconnected from my body during this time in my life already, but something shifted inside me after the abortion. It took something human out of me. Even though sex had always been painful for me, I suddenly stopped being able to force myself to do it. The thought of it made me feel sick with guilt. I kept running.

In 2015, I had a surgery that resulted from months and months of pain that was building again, worse than it had been in years, plaguing my body each day like clockwork. After the surgery, the symptoms didn't let up. If anything, they got worse. I told my doctor this in a very weak moment, sitting in his office, exhausted, confused, afraid. He explained to me that I can never expect his surgeries to fix me. He told me I had a condition that no one could fix.

He explained that it was devastating that so few people – so few doctors – understood the condition. That so few medical professionals understood its symptoms, or knew how debilitating it could be.

This lack of understanding of the legitimacy of the disease is the reason I still pull taxis over in the street and pay them to let me lie down for twenty minutes, to calm myself, to let the painkillers I have just taken sink into my body; all to avoid ever having to take a day off. To avoid ever needing to explain myself. Until a sustainable treatment or cure is developed, regular surgeries are my only option.

Multiple studies have now connected severe cases of endometriosis to the physiological effects of sexual trauma. But I didn't know that at the time of my diagnosis; I hadn't even accepted that I had been assaulted. I was still so far from getting better.

In among all of this, I slowly learned to accept my chronic illness but I was entirely dissociated from its cause. Once, in hospital, I was reading *The Empathy Exams* again and I was struck by Jamison's description of her anger at her own difficult medical situation. She wrote of her doctor:

> Dr M. became a villain because my story didn't have one.

I identified so strongly with those words that I cried when I read them. I thought of all the misplaced anger and hurt I felt at the fact that I was sick, that I wasn't getting better. That I would never get better. I imagined myself yelling at all the doctors who couldn't fix me, demonizing them because my story had no demons.

Except that it did. My story had a villain, but I was too afraid to face him. My mind had erased him from the narrative because the thought of him was unbearable. I thought, in that moment, lying in the hospital bed, thinking of all the villains my story lacked, that this confusion was the greatest indignity.

What I didn't realize then was that the indignity was far greater than I knew: the world had the answer to who had caused this pain, but it had kept it from me. Just like the memory itself, the truth of the connection between severe physical trauma and chronic illness was hidden.

This conceit made a spluttering fool out of me.

Later in 2015, in mid-November, I found myself,

once again, in the emergency department of a Sydney hospital, doubled over in agony and shaking from head to foot. The doctors on call decided to do an MRI to check for inflammation of the bowel. They found that a section of my small intestine was markedly inflamed.

That night I was diagnosed with Crohn's disease. I was put on a course of IV steroids and spent the next week in hospital. My body, it seemed, was in full-scale revolt. Still, it did not occur to me to think or speak of my assault. So, in my mind, my story remained untethered and devoid of appropriately directed cause.

What I would have given, in those moments, to know that my story could have a villain – a narrative – if only I were brave enough to see it. What I would have given to know there was someone to blame. That he was there somewhere, hiding in the darkest corners of my mind. That his face is permanently etched into my memory even though I will never know his name.

I had spent the years following the rape running so far away from myself that I thought the memory could not catch me. My life was an abstraction; I was a conscious being but I had no form, no boundaries. My body caused me so much pain that I refused to engage with it altogether. I only tended to it when it caused a crisis and gave me no choice. At all other times, I neglected it entirely.

I masked the pain with drugs that numbed me and refused to engage in any sensible long-term care for my condition. I could not accept that my new life was permanent. Gently, my doctors kept saying: This is not going to go away. You have to stop thinking you are going to get better. But I couldn't let go.

Instead of allowing myself to be vulnerable to the illness I could not wish away, I became defensive and bitter and angry. I rarely accepted help. I got sicker. In refusing to give in to my illness, I kept up as many aspects of my life as I could, trying desperately to play the part of the functional woman I had imagined I would turn out to be. I overcompensated. I took on too much. I got sicker.

I managed to construct a life this way. A deeply fulfilling one, and one for which I am very grateful. I had relationships and heartbreaks that I thought might kill me. I learned to drive. I discovered Adele. I got into university to study politics and I joined every club on campus.

I started reporting for the university newspaper. I moved to San Francisco to work with a team of investigative reporters. I built a fledgling career writing about gender for a national news site. I found editors who believed in me and who trusted me. A few years later I decided to do further study alongside my writing career so I started doing a law degree at night. I built a life that started to make sense to me. Sometimes I felt as though I had outrun myself.

By 2015, six years after my initial acute episode

of pain, vomiting and bleeding, I had two diagnoses: endometriosis and Crohn's disease. How unlucky, I thought at the time. Now I know the two are intimately connected: both are inflammatory disorders; both are a result of the malfunctioning of the autoimmune system. Studies now show that both can, in some instances, be connected to the long-term physical effects of untreated sexual trauma.

And here's the other thing about the medical records. They reported what I know now to be telltale signs of untreated trauma: consistent pain, an overactive inflammatory response, extreme distress and anxiety pre- and post-surgery, a problem with drinking too much to dull my pain and/or anxiety about pain, tremors.

To my twenty-six-year-old self, having now read countless books and attended hundreds of hours of therapy about the physiological symptoms of trauma and listened to lecture after lecture after lecture from the best trauma specialists in the world, it is so clear to me that I was presenting to emergency as a traumatized young woman whose unspeakable story, held deep in her blood and her bones, was beginning to show up on her skin. Whose body was trying to say something her mind could not.

If someone – anyone – had intervened at that stage, I might not now have two lifelong illnesses to contend with. But they didn't intervene because I had finally achieved the thing I'd always wanted: to them, I was invisible. My body was screaming the answer but no one was listening to it. Not even me.

For years I blamed doctors for not making the connection. I thought if someone had asked the right question, I might have been spared. But that was never true. It was just easier that way.

The truth is that one doctor did ask me if I had been raped. It was 2010, not long after I got sick, and I was being tested for Crohn's disease. He asked the question, and somehow I found myself telling him the story. It was the first time I had ever told it, out loud, from start to finish. I told him every detail. Once I started I couldn't stop. He looked deeply concerned and tried to respond but I didn't let him.

As soon as I'd finishing telling the story, I realized what I had done: that I had given myself away. The panic of that realization was unbearable. I couldn't take back the words so I, quite literally this time, ran away. I reached for the door and ran down the hallway to the elevators, and when I got to street level I kept running. I was hysterical, sobbing, crying, wishing I could disappear. Eventually, a taxi driver pulled over and asked if I was okay, and he drove me home. It was 10.30 a.m. but I got straight into bed and lay in a dark room for hours, punishing myself, wondering what had come over me, what on earth could have made me feel it was okay to tell the truth about my life.

The doctor called me every week for a month but I never spoke to him again. He tried everything he could to help me, but I wouldn't let him.

By far the most dangerous element of my assault was the fact that I lived in a world where it was unspeakable. I knew, as soon as it happened, without ever being told, that I must say nothing. Indignity is painful but silence is a prison.

What I now know is that no doctor would have been able to help me while I was trapped by silence and shame. The need to keep my secret was more powerful than anything else. Silence mattered more to me than my body, my health, even my life. I had always thought that the violence of this experience had been swift and obvious, a Swiss army knife and a bruised ribcage, but I was wrong. The far greater loss was invisible and insidious. It was the compulsion I felt every day to say nothing. It was not the terror of a bottle smashed over ceramic but the steady, everyday shame that followed. It was every tiny signal – in films, in conversations with friends, in music, in politics, in language – that made me believe this was my fault. It was a death by a thousand paper cuts.

The most important thing that was taken from me was the ability to say something, and with it, the ability to ask for help. This is a theft from which I will never recover.

But it is also more than a theft; it is an act of

violence itself. Trauma studies have now proven that abdominal surgeries can themselves cause symptoms of post-traumatic stress disorder (PTSD). Although the patient is unconscious, the body registers the intrusion and, depending on the person's predisposition to PTSD symptoms, the surgery itself can be a form of trauma. So in a truly cruel irony, my inability to voice my trauma led me to do diagnostic surgery after diagnostic surgery, each time causing further re-traumatization.

Since being diagnosed with endometriosis and Crohn's, I have had to undergo five surgeries to clear out the disease. Each of these was profoundly invasive. A disease caused by trauma for which the only known treatment causes trauma.

This is to say nothing of the fact that for a person with undiagnosed post-traumatic stress disorder, surgeries are particularly distressing because of the result of anaesthesia: the way you wake up from the surgery completely helpless, right back in that echoey bathroom with tall walls and a locked door and the glass and the tiles and the smell of whiskey.

To me, the most devastating part of gaining an understanding of the lifelong physical impacts of trauma is that they are unnecessary. Gratuitous. If trauma is treated immediately, full recovery is possible. Almost all of the long-term effects can be prevented.

This means, more often than not, the permanent impacts of trauma are reserved only for those with unspeakable stories. This strikes me as both one of the most catastrophic human tendencies and, simultaneously, one of the easiest to fix, which perhaps just makes the heartbreak worse still.

IV

A truth was being revealed to me: that I had always tried to attach myself to the light of other people, that I had never had any light of my own. I experienced myself as a kind of shadow.

Zadie Smith, *Swing Time*

DISAPPEARANCES

On 2 January 2018, a mentor and I were playing Cluedo with her young children, and she passed me a note asking me to give myself a score out of ten based on how much I agreed with the following statements:

I am a good person
I am selfish
I deserve to be happy

The kids accused us of cheating. I handed the note back:

I am a good person 2/10
I am selfish 9/10
I deserve to be happy 2/10

She handed it back and left a scrawled note next to them saying: This is not your voice. Whose voice is it?

I stared at the note. The voice of violation. The voice that tells you that you are worthless. I know now that one of the effects of untreated trauma on the body and mind is to make us ashamed; to make us believe that we are, and always will be, people to whom terrible things happen – people who deserve to be hunted.

This is put best in Meera Atkinson's *Traumata*:

Shame is often transmitted, paradoxically, by shameless acts, acts in which one person's avoidance of shame demands another carry it.

She says of the man who abused her: 'I was ashamed for him yet it was not my shame.'

The voice telling me I did not deserve to be happy was one that had been transmitted to me by a savage, shameless act. The decision of an unrepentant man who will never feel ashamed of his actions. So I am condemned to carry the shame for him, and I have. For so long, I have.

It is not my shame.

When I think now about the long therapeutic process of learning to manage that shame, I can't help but think of this moment as the moment I started to realize that perhaps this wasn't a fixed part of me.

That's not your voice. Whose voice is it?

Unlearning shame is one of the most difficult parts of trauma recovery, but it is possible. When I think back to the time when shame had a tyrannical hold over my life, unnamed and not yet recognized as something that did not belong to me, I think of a stanza from a poem by Megan Falley, called 'Holy Thank You for Not', one that I loved at the time but did not understand the prescience of:

Once you heard that Shame is the closest thing to Death.
Once you said *you* in a poem when you were too ashamed to say *I have wished to give my life back to my mother*
In a long dark box.

Shame really is the closest thing to death.

In the course of my recovery I have thought a lot about the nature of shame. How it is forced upon us by others; how it feels so personal but never belonged to us in the first place.

Once, sitting on a plane on my way to visit my sister and her new life in London, I stumbled upon a lecture by social scientist Brené Brown about the difference between shame and guilt, and it felt as though some fundamental truth about myself crystallized in one fell swoop.

Guilt and shame, she explained, are profoundly different emotions. Guilt is the feeling that you have done something bad; shame is the feeling that you *are* bad. Guilt is internally constructed, based on our knowledge of ourselves and the recognition that our behaviour has deviated from that self; shame, on the other hand, is given to us by others. Shame is inorganic.

Guilt says, I made a mistake.

Shame says, I am a mistake.

Guilt requires us to recognize that we have acted in a way that we regret, in a way that is out of character. This process is impossible for those who live with shame: for us, shame *is* our character.

There is no sense in which we can act in a manner that is 'unlike ourselves' when we have no 'self' to speak of. Shame devours us from the inside out and leaves us empty: with no solid form, no edges, no boundaries, no structure.

This is known in trauma literature as a lack of 'self-leadership'. When a person's development is defined by, or interrupted by, violence, they become unable to develop a clear sense of self. This is because their interiority – their capacity to make decisions, to understand what they want and don't want in the world – can only develop in an environment of safety. It is only in safe places that they can look inward. When their lives are beset by violence, they do not have that luxury.

As a traumatized child, you become accustomed to having to protect yourself, which means having a razor-sharp awareness of everything around you. You have to be able to sense danger from a mile away. You become hyper-vigilant.

Once you experience this fight, flight, freeze response, particularly in a truly life-threatening situation, it lives on in your body and resurfaces again and again in everyday life. Scientists call this a false positive bias: once you learn how perilous the world can be, you will interpret every single moment of ambiguity as danger.

Hyper-vigilance is very sensible from an evolutionary perspective. But when trauma becomes chronic and hyper-vigilance becomes a way of life, it is this very survival instinct that ironically keeps us from living in any meaningful sense of the word. We become a bundle of reactions, with no internal core, moulded together by circumstance. A precarious glue. The only sense of self we can find is the one we see reflected back to us by others. We hunt for clues in others' behaviour as to the type of person we are. This delivers to us a funny kind of magic trick: we are able to construct a new self from one moment to the next depending on our audience. Like the tree falling in the proverbial forest, we feel that if no-one is watching, we won't really exist at all.

And so, as I grew older, I learned to curate different versions of myself around different people. I learned to reflect back to each person their favourite parts of themselves. I learned that this is the surest way to win approval. I was no longer a girl. I was a mirror.

I gave whatever the audience asked for. I took nothing because I had no self to nourish. I built a personality out of my unending capacity to respond to the needs of others.

Once I was sitting in a close friend's apartment texting a boy about meeting up later that night. He was so clearly keeping his options open, not even remotely interested in me as a person. I kept saying to my friend, I wonder when he'll text so I know what I'm doing tonight. She looked bemused at this prospect: What do you actually want to do? I had no answer and we sat in silence. I had no earthly idea what I *wanted* to do. It's not something I ever thought about.

Once I lied about desperately needing a glass of water, even though one was being offered to me, on a humid Sydney summer's day because I was so afraid of inconveniencing anyone. It's almost as if I was scared that if I said yes to the offer, they might notice that I was there.

Once I lied to a nurse in an emergency department about needing more morphine because she looked so busy and I didn't want to cause her additional stress. The truth was I needed the morphine. Badly. But that was an internal need, and I had learned that external cues must always take priority.

This notion of a lack of self-leadership, a lack of interiority, of a stable personality, is connected to our deeply held belief that there is something putrid inside of us; something poisonous and toxic and immutable. We become people-pleasers as a way of ensuring that no-one ever looks at us too closely. We conceal ourselves because we are so ashamed that if we are seen, the rotten core will be seen too. It is an ongoing act of disappearance.

I found myself dependent not only on the approval of others but also on external symbols of success: good marks and gold medals and perfect report cards. I stayed up all night perfecting every piece of homework I submitted because I knew if I got a good mark, I'd have something to hang my hat on. Look, I would be able to tell myself, this is me.

It is shame that silences us, and spreads our silence to others. It is a deathly contagion. If shame is erasure, then its opposite must surely be our insistence on structure: on shape, on form. It must surely be a relentless insistence on being seen. On telling the truth.

I looked down at my mentor's note again. As well as her question, she had also crossed out my answers and replaced them with her own, so now the note read:

I am a good person 9/10
I am selfish 3/10
I deserve to be happy 10/10

For weeks, I carried that note in my pocket wherever I went, I tried to get serious about treating my post-traumatic stress disorder.

I was in my final year of law school and was desperately trying to hold it together. I had a job I loved but found myself unable to keep up with it. I was determined to run far enough away from my illnesses that I would never have to face their common cause. I was a girl who desperately wanted to get better, who secretly knew the way out, but couldn't accept it. Couldn't accept that getting better would mean disclosure, would mean breaking the most important promise she had ever made to herself.

I hated my body because it had caused me so much pain and because so many doctors had convinced me it was untrustworthy. I distrusted it deeply, I wished it would disappear. I wanted a new one. But instead, in that decade between my assault and my recovery, with all the surgeries and doctors and question marks, I simply left my body altogether. I only acknowledged its pain when it was physically crippling me; the rest of the time I numbed it with heavy painkillers, alcohol and potent self-hatred. By the time I was nearing my final law exams, my physical and mental health were deteriorating rapidly.

It's strange that the body's dissociative fight, flight or freeze response can be so destructive, because its evolutionary purpose is a very sensible one: it is designed to protect us from experiencing the pain of our dying moments; moments the brain does not think it will ever have to fold into any kind of narrative because it does not think it will live to tell the story at all.

Unfortunately, this means that the act of living through these moments is a subversion with which the brain cannot fully cope, and it tortures us physically as it tries to make sense of it. This is why they call us survivors.

I struggled through preparations for an important trial, I wrote a law thesis and tried to squeeze in freelance journalism on the side. I was distracting myself. I was still unable to accept the truth of my illness, and of my assault, plagued by nightmares and memories that were closing in on me like a pack of wolves.

One night in late 2017, I found myself going home with a man I had already had a non-consensual sexual encounter with. I knew he was aggressive. I told him I was in pain and couldn't have sex, and he pretended to be okay with it.

A dedicated friend, one of the only people who knew what I was going through, tried to stop me from leaving with him. When that failed, she texted me three times while I was in the cab to tell me it was okay just to go home, I didn't have to go through with it. I thanked her, and meant it, but stayed in the Uber with him anyway. Frozen.

Sometimes, under an extreme degree of traumatic

stress, the body becomes so overwhelmed that it simply gives itself over to whatever is threatening it. In this bizarre counter-evolutionary state, we put ourselves in harm's way to numb the feeling of helplessness.

This has been noted in volcanic eruptions, when animals become so overwhelmed by the stress of the situation that they run into the lava. Once, a volcano erupted on an island off the coast of Indonesia and several species were tracked heading towards the danger, including sea lions, who had a perfectly safe means of escape by simply staying underwater and swimming away. Instead, they swam into the volcano and let it burn them alive.

So there I was, sitting in the Uber, watching my dear friend's worried text messages arrive one after the other, knowing as she did that I was swimming, full-tilt, into the volcano.

When we got back to his house, he insisted on having sex despite my pain. In my head I was screaming in pain and distress, but my body was limp and my voice had jumped out of my throat and hidden somewhere. I distinctly remember feeling as though I was floating above my body again, watching myself relive a waking nightmare. I felt no pain in those moments. I just watched. I waited.

When it was over I returned to my body and the pain was unbearable. I wanted so badly to get up and leave, but the pain in my stomach was so sharp that I could not move my legs. I willed them to muster the strength but they refused.

I lay there and allowed the shame to envelop me, and I hoped I would somehow disappear. I wanted no one to see or hear from me again. In that moment, I wished for the mercy of a raging volcano; the swiftness with which it would destroy me and leave no trace of me behind.

The next day I went home and tried to pretend it hadn't happened, but when I turned on the shower, my wrists ached from the way he'd held them down. My legs shook for days. I lay in my room and wondered how I could have done something so reckless despite knowing how badly it would hurt me.

I didn't know, then, about those sea lions.

But this was more than a confused evolutionary reaction to danger; it was a form of self-harm. I didn't put myself in that situation in spite of how much it would hurt me, I did so because I knew that it would. I was so ashamed of my past that I punished myself by recreating it.

Trauma research has proven the desire for 're-enactment' in survivors. This means that people who have been traumatized and unable to escape develop a neuropathology in which they become attracted to situations that replicate their traumatic experience.

We do this because in trauma our brain's fight-or-flight response proves ineffectual and we become helpless. What this does to the body is create an extremely high level of energy in the muscles and the blood, ready for escape, but this energy is never discharged. So, physically and psychologically, we seek out, again and again, situations in which we might be able to discharge that energy and relieve ourselves from the physical damage it causes us.

We seek to re-enact the trauma because we want to prove that it can end differently, because the body is evolutionarily conditioned to attempt to fix its mistakes for the benefit of the species. The problem is that the freeze response is not one we are meant to survive, so biologically, it is not well adapted to the process of re-enactment.

This condemns traumatized people to a life in which danger seems to be ever-present. We internalize this. In Hanya Yanagihara's A Little Life, her protagonist, Jude, is an adult man who was sexually abused as a child and who finds himself in abusive situations in adulthood too. The character ponders:

The axiom of equality states that x always equals x: it assumes that if you have a conceptual thing named x, that it must always be equivalent to itself, that it has a uniqueness about it, that it is in possession of something so irreducible that we must assume it

is absolutely, unchangeably equivalent to itself for
all time, that its very elementalness can never be
altered . . .

The person I was will always be the person I am, he
realizes . . . a person who inspires disgust, a person
meant to be hated.

In Jude's mind, this mathematical formula represents
an entire life: x will always equal x. No matter how
far you run from yourself, no matter how fast, you
will always have the same irreducible, rotten core.
When the character is much older and in a physically
abusive relationship with yet another predatory man,
his partner throws him down the stairs and as he hears
his shoulder crack on the cement below, he thinks to
himself: x equals x. x equals x. x equals x.

I re-enacted my sexual assault by constantly exposing
myself to men who would force themselves into me,
by ignoring the freeze and the pain. I sought out
relationship after relationship in which my consent
didn't matter because my body was conditioned to
replay that same scene, over and over, to dress-rehearse
death just to prove it could survive.

My mind, confused by a hyper-vigilant sense of
danger, was putting me in harm's way. My body
screamed in revolt but I kept going. At the same time
as reconstructing these moments of helplessness, I was

falling prey to my mind's desperate desire to escape by self-destruction. I constantly found new ways to disappear.

I built up an arsenal of destructive behaviours that would satisfy the part of me that wanted to be invisible but that would not put me at risk of serious self-harm. I chased men who thought nothing of me just to prove to myself that I was unworthy. I chased away people who offered me kindness for exactly the same reason. I never occurred to me that I might be the author of my own disappointment.

Once trauma finds you it does not let you go. And so we re-traumatize ourselves, believing we are rotten because we are the type of people to whom bad things happen, when in fact it is the living, breathing memory of the first bad thing that keeps sending us back, again and again and again, into the volcano.

It is a self-fulfilling prophecy.

Every time I had sex during that last semester, the pain would become so bad I often had to stay in bed for days; sometimes I even had to take myself to hospital because of the profound effect the invasion had on my body. And yet I kept doing it, kept chasing the shame and hurt I would feel after confirming to myself that I would never get over what happened to me.

When I look back on this time now, it seems as though this was when the memory of the attack truly started to close in on me. I started having more detailed dreams about it. My pain became unbearable and almost constant. After sex I would vomit for hours to try to purge myself of the piercing sensation it left me with.

And so it was that the shame I had always felt about being a sick woman, a failed woman, was compounded by my first conscious thoughts that I was also a rape victim.

I made it to work at my law firm most days, but the nights were the worst part: too uncomfortable to sleep, too determined to turn up at work the next day to take proper painkillers, too exhausted by my illness to lose another night's rest. In daylight I appeared as though I was coping, but it was during these nights that I realized the structure I had built of myself was crumbling; I could feel it breaking somewhere inside me.

The pain kept getting worse, the vomiting, the shaking. The memories were catching up with me and I was losing the momentum I needed to keep running.

The pain became unbearable and more difficult to hide. I lost seven kilos in four weeks. I was inexplicably throwing up half of what I ate, and I started shaking so much I had to get friends to help me put on make-up. I started missing lectures and days at work. My blood pressure dropped and I started passing out at random intervals.

My tremors and weight loss became conspicuous enough that a close friend asked how I was doing. I told him I had lost control of my hands and I was collapsing regularly without warning. He looked concerned, and told me to call the doctor. I nodded, absent-mindedly, and stared into my glass of wine.

Why won't you call the doctor? he asked.

In that moment I was so weak that I made an admission I had never allowed myself to make before, even in my own head.

I'm scared.

He held my hands and told me it would be okay. As we stood there, in his kitchen, I felt something I never expected to feel: I felt relieved that I had admitted to him that I was afraid. I felt relieved that he held my hands and I felt relieved that I let him hold them. I felt cared for. It was February 2018, and it was the first time I thought I might be ready to ask for help. I turned twenty-six later that week. I didn't feel there was anything to celebrate.

About a week later I left work mid-morning and collapsed on my bed. I woke up eight hours later, backpack and shoes still on, disoriented and afraid. I woke up in a daze, unable to move my arms and unable to feel my legs. The pain in my abdomen was blinding. Every joint felt so inflamed that I could not move a muscle. I had a law exam to prepare for but I couldn't stay awake.

It was early March 2018, only a few months shy of my graduation. I thought I could get through it. But I had pushed my body so far that I had once again become completely helpless. I had been swimming straight into the volcano and I hadn't even realized it.

I reached over and swallowed some codeine so I could return to unconsciousness.

The next time I woke up was almost twenty-four hours later. I wasn't sure if I'd overdosed or if my body really was starting to shut down. I called an Uber and went to the other side of Sydney to my GP. By the time I got there, I was barely conscious. My blood pressure was dangerously low. The doctor discovered I had lost five kilos since being weighed two weeks earlier.

She called a taxi and sent me to hospital. The doctors wanted to put me on another course of steroids but I refused. A dietician came to see me and prescribed me a powerful supplement powder, telling me that I had a window of two to three days in which to return to a normal weight before my body would adapt to a state of malnutrition.

When the doctors were trying to impress upon me the urgency of this situation, they kept using words like 'collapse' and 'shutdown'.

I notice now that these terms are used frequently in trauma studies. These doctors, of course, were not using these terms in this way. They were simply describing what they saw in me: a physical form that had degraded to the point of near-total dysfunction. But to me it seems important that these states are similar to those experienced in trauma; it betrays just how cunning the mind can be. No matter how far you run, no matter how fast, it catches you, and places you right back where you started.

I have always tried hard to be a generous person, but at that time in my life I found myself being ruthlessly unkind to just about everyone around me. I said and thought cruel things about people who had never deserved cruelty. I was merciless in my approximation of the people who failed to help me, even though I continued to fail to help myself.

I hated everyone because I could not bear the weight of how much I hated myself. It was as if I had to apportion the loathing before it buried me alive. Or perhaps I just became so practised at being cruel to myself that it spread to others. Perhaps anger bleeds.

My weight dropped to 43 kilos and I looked skeletal. Another act of disappearance.

As I stood on the hospital-grade scale one morning when the doctors were desperately trying to see if I was gaining weight, I looked at the flashing digital number, 43, and had a sudden memory of seeing that number on a scale once before.

Years earlier, about five years after my sexual assault, I developed an eating disorder and began starving myself and throwing up when I broke my own rules. I hated my body so much I could barely leave the house. So I started to break it down, to destroy it, to diminish it until I could barely see it at all.

I used to run the shower while I threw up my lunch, so my housemates wouldn't notice.

I got down to 43 kilos just before I realized how unwell I was and decided to get help. There it was, that same number again, all these years later.

One way or another, the body keeps the score.

By late March my tremors were becoming uncontrollable. I invited a new friend over for tea and accidentally poured boiling water all over my bare hand because I could not control my fingers. I'm so clumsy, I said to him, shaking my head.

The people closest to me were alarmed: I was skeletal and my tremors were alarmingly obvious. I no longer had the stoicism about my pain that they had all become so accustomed to. I started having long episodes, days on end, of inflammatory joint pain so bad that I could hardly move a bone in my body. I just lay there, staring at the ceiling, hoping it would end, not caring how.

The ulcers in my mouth caused by Crohn's flares meant that I couldn't eat solid food because my mouth filled with blood each time I tried. I started eating soup in bed for every meal. Every time I brushed my teeth, no matter how gently, it cracked open all the wounds in my mouth, and after about twenty seconds I would be brushing my teeth with my own blood. So I stopped brushing my teeth. Then I stopped showering. Then I stopped getting out of bed at all.

I took extended sick leave from work and was in

and out of hospital, while they monitored my weight and tried to figure out why nothing was working. I kept insisting on being discharged because every hospital admission felt like a brand-new failure. I knew I was too sick to be at home, especially in a Sydney shared house where no one was attuned to my comings and goings, but I couldn't stand to admit that I needed to stay in hospital. Concerned doctors in fancy suits argued with me but eventually let me go home, only to find me back in the ward a few days later.

One day I went to my GP to check in with her and after weighing me, she noticed that I was still rapidly losing weight.

You need to be in hospital, she said.

This is not safe.

I thanked her for the advice but told her that one of my best friends was getting married that Friday outside of Sydney and I wouldn't miss it for the world. She looked at me as if I was crazy, but I meant it. I loved my friends deeply and I wanted so badly to share their joy with them.

Even though a huge part of me wanted to die, I wanted to be at the wedding more. I wanted to at least stay alive until then.

I made it through the ceremony and I even made it to the after-party, but by then I really felt I was in danger. That morning I had been so desperate not to cause a fuss, not to make this happy day about my illness, and yet by the end of the night, I didn't care if I died on the dance floor. I hadn't met this version of myself – so selfish, so inconsiderate – until that night.

That night the pain was so bad as I lay there that I really thought it might kill me. This is it, I thought.

I remember feeling guilty about the two men I'd only met a few months before who were in the room with me, who would have to find my body the next morning. I felt terrible for my friend, one of my closest and dearest friends, whose wedding would be forever marred by my grand and dramatic failure. But for the first time in my life, that guilt was eclipsed: I just wanted it to be over.

A few days later I was lying in bed making plans to commit suicide. It seems cruel that your mind convinces you that you want to die after your body has done so much to keep you alive.

I lay thinking about how I would do it, how I could minimize the inconvenience to the men I lived with. I have never been religious but I found myself laying there, hugging my knees, repeating the same phrase over and over again.

It's a phrase I learned from Margaret Atwood's *The Handmaid's Tale*. The main character, June Osborne, explains the etymology of the word 'mayday'. It is an anglicized version of the French phrase, 'm'aidez'. It means: help me.

I found myself repeating this in my head over and over as if it were a prayer of some kind. It had a rhythm and it didn't stop for hours. It went like this: first, the commonly used English version, then the French, then the English translation, repeated three times.

Mayday.
M'aidez.
Help me.
Help me.
Help me.

It was after that day that I started taking seriously the possibility that my physical disability was, or could be, a consequence of the assault. It was then I realized that if I properly started to understand the relationship between the two, I might finally find some peace.

I had tried everything I could to get better, and nothing had worked. I was finally ready to try anything. Even the one thing I swore I would never do.

Realizing, after how serious I was about suicide that day, just how close I had come to letting this memory drown me, I kept thinking about another line from *The Handmaid's Tale*. June, the protagonist, who is captured in a theocratic nightmare in which she is exposed to ritual rape on a regular basis, says to the reader: I intend to survive.

It is this line that made me realize the true significance of the term 'survivors'. It does not refer only to surviving the traumatic incident itself, but the everyday terror that follows. The days and weeks and years of indignity that follow. Some days I think that part came closer to killing me than the man with the knife did. But I intend to survive.

V

This home is what I came into this world with,
Was the first home,
Will be the last home,
You can't take it.

Rupi Kaur, 'I'm taking my body back'

RECOVERY

When I was fifteen, I was attacked by a grown man with a knife. I was a child. I was an athlete. I was fearless. Nothing mattered as much to me as the way my body worked, the incredible things it could do, the way it could fly like no one else's. I was consumed by the audacity of self-belief. And then I came crashing down to earth. Into the gutter where I belonged, where I was powerless, where no one would notice me.

The body I felt so comfortable in, the home I had built for myself, became a battlefield. Something that had always made sense to me became entirely opaque. I didn't understand the way my muscles moved, I didn't understand the way my bones ached, I didn't understand why I had lost my balance.

I was covered in bruises and something had cracked

inside me. In moments, I lost the thing I had spent my whole life building. I became a visitor in my own skin. I ran and ran and it took me ten years to find my way back. It took me ten years even to try.

But slowly I realized that getting better meant being brave enough to occupy my body again. To be brave enough to feel the pain of it, the weakness of it, to bear witness to how broken it had become. It was only once I started to do that that my body and I started to understand each other again.

The psychologist Elizabeth Waites describes trauma as 'injury to mind or body that requires structural repair'. I had spent so long pretending I hadn't been hurt, but I had. I needed structural repair and nothing less than that would help me.

In my first job as a journalist, I covered issues of women's safety – primarily sexual assault and domestic violence. When I was twenty-three I reported a story about some of the physical impacts of rape. I went back to my notes from the piece and started following my own leads – a trail I had left myself long before I knew where it would take me. I spent whole evenings scouring the internet to try to figure out who could help me. I started reading books about post-traumatic stress. I investigated its treatment, its telltale signs. When I had read enough to accept that it was possible this was part of my story, I called therapists and physios and specialists and told them I needed to see someone urgently.

To the tune of looped hold music, I silently begged for someone to answer before I changed my mind.

I found a medical psychotherapist who has supported me more than I could have imagined. He has led me through sessions of a painful treatment called Eye Movement Desensitization and Reprocessing: an intense therapy using rapid eye movements that forces the brain to recall a memory in a safe environment, after which it can be processed as something already lived through. This therapy allows the past and the present to finally let go of each other.

I learned to identify the sensations that enliven the fragments of the memory in my mind – the sound of a glass bottle smashed accidentally at a house party, the smell of a particular mix of whiskey and cigarettes on a man's breath, the echo you hear when you inadvertently knock an elbow against a wall in a public bathroom. The devil, it turns out, really is in the details.

I found a sex therapist who has dedicated herself to the sexual health aspects of my care. During my first appointment with her I told her about my assault and she told me I was brave. I cried. She asked me who else knew. Hardly anyone, I said. She looked heartbroken.

You have been holding this assault in your body, all on your own, for over ten years, she said after a few moments.

I didn't know enough about the physiology of

trauma back then to know what she meant, but now I do, and I am so grateful to her for recognizing what had happened to me months before I would be able to recognize it myself.

She taught me about a condition called vaginismus, which is when the vaginal and pelvic floor muscles become so frozen from pain that they stop functioning altogether. She also told me about the way an attack can cause the body to shut off nerve endings in particular parts of the body altogether to prevent pain, as a kind of ever-present analgesic.

Together, we worked to try to make me feel safe enough to inhabit my body again, to tell the parts of me that had run away that it was okay to come back. That I would listen to them when they were in pain. That I would be gentle this time. She taught me to do exercises with hot packs and cold packs on different parts of my body, so they could get used to experiencing physical sensations again.

During one session, we did an exercise called 'waking up the hands'. She gave me an object and asked me to hold it and pay attention to how it felt in my hands, underneath my fingers. What did my fingers like the most on this object, she asked. I asked my fingers what they liked, which parts of the object they wanted to touch, and I listened when they answered. I think it was the first time in over a decade that my mind and my body were reunited.

My gynaecological surgeon referred me to a highly skilled women's health physiotherapist who specialized in dealing with the physical effects of severe sexual assault. She has been using internal and external manual therapy techniques to release the muscle dysfunction this experience left me with. Through breathing exercises, stretching, mindfulness, pelvic floor 'down training' and massage, I have been retraining my body not to freeze up every time it is touched.

This process has been painful and exhausting, but it's working.

My physiotherapist specializes in sexual assault and during our third session, she examined my genital muscles. This is an internal examination. Lying there, feeling comfortable with her, I did not dissociate. The months of learning to reinhabit my body were working and instead of floating away, I stayed there, and I listened. Without this dissociation – as soon as I had learned to allow my body to tell me what it was feeling – every single touch in that part of my body was excruciating. She tried to examine my pelvic floor muscles by putting a finger inside me and the pain was so sharp – like a Swiss army knife – that I cried and cried and we had to stop.

If this was how my body reacted to the slightest touch, I couldn't imagine what I had put it through while I was gone.

On days like this, when the true cost of my assault

became apparent to me, I wanted to rewind. To return to the body of the girl who had not acknowledged the gravity of her experience.

I imagined myself approaching one of those big red signs on Australian single-lane highways that says: WRONG WAY, GO BACK.

But every time I came close to giving up, I thought of the comforting words my best friend offers me when she notices that I'm in trouble: the only way out of it is through it.

So I kept going.

As I was trying to heal, I learned to turn all of my energy inward. I spent hours and hours alone. I never knew who or what might upset me in public, so I perfected the art of leaving the party without saying goodbye. I would slip away before anyone could see me break down, slink into the safety of an Uber, comforted only by the unexpected kindness of the stranger behind the wheel. In the back seat, I would have the uneasy sense of being both frozen and melting: half terror, half tears. I would call a trusted friend and ask them to meet me at home and stay with me until I fell asleep.

I moved into a house with one of my oldest friends and I finally felt calm again. I stopped going out and drinking too much and learned to spend hours and hours alone with my thoughts, no matter how painful they were. I still wanted to die but I was getting better at resisting the pull to act on that feeling.

I started getting massages once a week to relax my muscles and to help them recover from the intensive physical therapy I was undergoing. I started stretching every day to wake up my muscles to movement after years of being frozen still by fear and pain.

I promised my body I would not subject it to sex until it was ready. This is a promise I have kept, and my world is so much safer for it.

I forced myself to spend an hour every day writing poems, no matter how clumsy or heavy-handed they were, as a way of grounding myself. I learned to meditate, and slowly, I regained the mental stillness I used to deploy so skilfully on the gym floor.

After years of hating and avoiding doctors, I told myself I must go to every single appointment. No excuses. And I did. Each Friday, I would see all my specialists, one after the other. No matter how much I didn't want to. No matter how scared I was. No matter how exhausting my recovery had become. I kept showing up, week after week.

I went on antidepressants to help with the suicidal thoughts enlivened by reliving the memories. I started taking muscle relaxants to help my body calm down. I started eating turmeric every day to settle my body's inflammatory system. For the first time in my life, I was good at taking care of myself. I got better at accepting help when it was offered to me.

I started reading books again. When I needed a

break from the memories, I would read whole novels in one sitting. I sat in the bath for hours, listening to my favourite poems on repeat, lying motionless until the water grew cold and my fingers turned to raisins.

Crohn's disease and endometriosis are lifelong illnesses. They can be managed, but not cured. This is a theft for which I will never be compensated. Living with that reality has been a difficult process, but I have come to accept it. It is no longer a source of anger, or fear, or resentment. It just *is*. It took more than ten years, but I have finally released myself from the need to pretend this assault hadn't happened to me, hadn't changed me. I have finally relinquished the fantasy that I can go back to the body of the girl I used to be.

Everything I've ever let go of has claw marks on it.

My recovery has not been easy. It has been slow, at times excruciatingly painful and demoralizing. But I'm making progress. I have finally placed this memory into the narrative of my life in a way that makes sense to me.

In one of her now-famous 'Dear Sugar' columns, Cheryl Strayed recounted the following anecdote when giving advice to a rape victim:

I have a friend who is twenty years older than me who was raped three different times over the course of her life . . . I asked her how she recovered from them, how she continued having healthy sexual relationships with men. She told me that at a certain point we get to decide who it is we allow to influence us. She said, 'I could allow myself to be influenced by three men who screwed me against my will or I could allow myself to be influenced by Van Gogh. I chose Van Gogh.'

When I read these words, I thought of all of the women writers who kept me company during the darkest moments of my recovery. The women whose strength pushed me ever on, convincing me that there was a world out there that was beautiful and kind and safe, and that it would be waiting for me when I was ready for it.

I thought of my favourite author, Elena Ferrante, and the way her stories of female friendship showed me that women can be soft and powerful; that tenderness and strength are not antithetical, but equivalent. It takes vulnerability and resilience for women like her protagonist, Elena Greco, to overcome their dangerous pasts and possess their own narratives, in all of their complexity. In all of their vulnerability.

I can choose to be influenced by a violent man in an abandoned bathroom or I can choose to be influenced by the strength and honesty of Elena.

A few months ago, I went to a ballet class for the first time in years. It was devastating to see how stiff my body had become in the years I'd neglected it, how profoundly damaged it was. But it was also an unparalleled joy to be reminded, even for a moment, of the feeling of being strong and powerful and poised and graceful and beautiful all at once.

I went to a private gymnastics lesson with one of the athletes I used to compete with. As she watched me relearn my tricks, she scanned her eyes over my body and I heard in her words the echo of every coach, every athlete and every judge I'd ever trained with. They had noticed the same things she was noticing now: my impressively high arches, my hyperextended knees, my stubborn hamstrings. She promised me everything would come back to me quickly, and it did. The memory of how to move like I used to was still there, in my muscles.

My body had kept everything in its rightful place, waiting for me to come back to it.

VI

Unlike stories, real life, when it has passed, inclines toward obscurity, not clarity.

Elena Ferrante, *The Story of the Lost Child*

A man I admired. A man who had hurt me, again and again and again.

Of course I already knew this. The part of me that froze in that moment was full of every memory of inappropriate contact he made with me; full of frozen moments during massages that went too far; frozen moments during cuddles that didn't feel right. He had crossed many boundaries that I had pretended to ignore but in this moment, I no longer could. He had groomed me for years; a fact I knew in my body, in my muscles, but had never accepted in my mind. In that moment, it felt as though the whole world would collapse. Instead, I did. I fell to the floor and sat there, frozen, crying, confused, in the middle of the condiments aisle.

Everything turned to glass and shattered: the fragments of my life, my childhood, lay strewn around me on the floor of Banana Joe's. My vision blurred. The shelves of jams and chutneys became fluid and every solid boundary around me dissolved.

I don't know how long I sat there. I don't know how many people asked me if I was okay, if I'd slipped on something. I don't know what happened next. I don't know how I got home but the next thing I knew I was lying in the bath, fantasizing about drowning myself, about how painful and difficult it would be, about how much I would deserve it, how sweet the relief would be when it ended, how maybe I could drown the vile part of myself that attracted abusers, again, and again, and again. The shame enveloped me like the bathwater and I stewed in it for hours.

I then had to rethink every formative aspect of my childhood; I had to transform a powerful young athlete into a victim. An easy target. Nothing made sense any more and I wanted to die more than I wanted to live with this revelation.

I have reached out to some of the gymnasts I used to train with. I am not the only one he hurt.

I know what you're thinking: gymnastics was the positive part of this story. How could she ruin that for us?

I know that's what you're thinking because that's exactly what I thought in those moments. But my duty to you is not to comfort you or provide you with a narrative that is clean and uncomplicated. My duty to you is to tell the truth. Because the truth matters, and telling the truth matters. Even when it is easier not to. Especially when it is easier not to.

And the truth is this: once you are vulnerable to trauma, once it gets its claws into you, it plays out again, and again, and again, like a broken record, until you confront it.

The truth is that other teenagers on that night in 2007 would have run away screaming at the first sign of coercion by an unknown male predator. Because I had been groomed as a child, I was adept at the freeze response, and I switched it on like a light when he took my hand and led me away. The truth is that my rape and my childhood abuse are not separate instances of bad luck; they are deeply and profoundly connected to one another. The truth is that if a frog is placed in boiling water it will jump straight out, but if it is placed in tepid water that is gradually boiled at an imperceptible pace, the animal – having proven at all other evolutionary junctures its capacity for survival – will boil alive.

The truth is, also, that gymnastics did make me powerful. It did give me a sense of embodiment that most teenage girls never get to feel. It did make me feel invincible, and it still does now, when I train. None of that was a lie; none of that is rendered untrue by the fact of my abuse. The two exist alongside each other, in a strange and uncomfortable union: the institution that made my body strong and powerful and autonomous as a teenager was the same one that primed me for the ultimate act of violation that would leave me physically disabled, forever.

The shame that kept me from reporting the childhood abuse is the same shame that kept me from voicing its sequel, and the same feeling that kept me from getting the help that I needed until it was almost too late.

In 1986, a young medical student named Larry Nassar joined the staff of USA Gymnastics as a trainer. While completing medical school, Larry ascended the ranks of the top gymnastics team's medical staff.

In 1996, he was appointed national medical coordinator for USA Gymnastics, a position he would occupy for eighteen years.

He trained some of the best athletes in the country. He was a mentor and a father figure as well as a doctor. His reputation was unassailable.

In 2017–2018, Larry Nassar was convicted and sentenced to 175 years in prison for the sexual abuse of gymnasts in his care. The court found that he has abused more than 260 women and girls. Under the guise of medical treatment, he would bring young girls alone into his treatment room and put his fingers inside them, inside their ten-, eleven-, twelve-year-old bodies. His penis was erect as he massaged them and as he violated them.

In a state of total freeze, they lay there and waited for it to end.

When Olympian McKayla Maroney was an athlete, Nassar gave her sleeping pills on an overseas flight they were taking to a competition. She woke up alone in a room with him, receiving one of his medical 'treatments'.

I thought I was going to die that night, she told a court eighteen years later.

She was fifteen at the time. When the abuse started, she was thirteen.

Chelsea Markham was ten when she was abused by Larry Nassar in one of his treatment sessions. The following year, she had a major fall at a competition. He was in the audience, she said later, and every time she saw him, she said she had flashbacks to the assault and lost her balance. It was the last time she would ever compete.

He hurt me, Chelsea told her mother in the car on the way back from the appointment during which she was molested by Nassar.

He put his fingers in me, she said.

But no one believed her. She quit gymnastics and never looked back. In 2009, Chelsea Markham committed suicide. Her mother blames Nassar's abuse for her death.

Alexis Moore and Olivia Cowan were each abused by Nassar for ten years.

Jennifer Rood Bedford was assaulted by Nassar on an operating table. She forced herself to say nothing.

I assumed something like what happened to me would only happen if I wanted it to, she said, years later.

Jennifer was a child, but she was old enough to know she would be blamed. Old enough to know she wouldn't be believed.

Madeleine Jones was eleven years old when Nassar began to abuse her.

I remember laying there frozen stiff on the table, utterly mortified, confused and scared, she said. Just like her body on the table, the words froze inside her

The realization that my fellow athletes were being abused in the same gyms, the same rooms, as I was, made me think about what would have happened if we'd told someone back then, in the early 2000s, about our abuse. And the answer seems clear: though I don't know for sure, I do wonder if it would have been the same thing that happened to Larry Nassar's victims, the ones who spoke up thirty years before his conviction. It's possible that we simply would not have been believed. That's the truth, the long and the short of it. It is such a simple fact, and such a complicated one. I am only just learning that those two things can be true at the same time.

What it also forced me to consider, for the first time in my life, was what would have happened if I had reported my rape to the police. I never, ever considered doing so. Honestly, the thought never crossed my mind because I so quickly decided to dedicate myself to pretending it never happened. I knew – intellectually – that someone, whoever he was, had committed a crime that night. I knew – intellectually – that I was his victim. I knew – intellectually – that I should stop him from hurting other teenage girls. But to do that would be to accept, to concede, that he had hurt *me*, and I wouldn't be ready to do that for another ten years.

So my rape went unreported, for the same reason so many sexual assaults do: I knew that shame could hurt more than the attack did. I knew that I lived in a world where the cost of speaking up could be much higher than any I had already paid. I had lost so much, and I was scared, and I was tired, and protecting myself from the blame of others was the only way I knew how to regain control.

I thought of the cross-examination. They could ask me why I didn't come forward earlier. Why was I out drinking on a Saturday when I was only fifteen? Why did I lie to my parents about where I was going that night? What did you expect would happen? they would ask.

To admit, again and again, to a stranger in front of a room full of other strangers, that this had happened to me, and then to have to insist that it had happened to me when I was accused of lying? That seemed unbearable in a way that pretending it hadn't happened didn't, so the choice between the two was easy.

Where is the evidence? They would ask.

Their search would turn up nothing. Any proof of my rape was washed down the drain of the shower on that night in 2007 as I sat on the floor, bleeding, crying, scrubbing myself clean. It faded along with the bruises he left on my chest and stomach. The ones I lied about. The ones I covered up as best I could.

I buried the evidence. All of it. Because I wanted to make sure no one ever found out that I was the kind of person this happened to.

Like the majority of rape defendants, the man with the Swiss army knife would likely be acquitted. His defence lawyer would talk about the family he probably has now – I imagine he would be about forty-five – and beg the jury not to let a woman with a decade-old allegation ruin the life he has built for himself. They would talk about his career. About how far he's come, about how sad it would be to take that all away from him.

What about my career? What about the Olympic gymnast I could have been? What about the small girl with the big smile and the relentless ambition? What about the writer, the girl who wrote tiny novels and poems but had her own story stolen from her? What about the lawyer, the one who wanted to change the world but can't sit up for more than a few hours at a time even on a good day?

The jury wouldn't hear anything about her. Except that she's a liar, a rotten thing. I would have to watch as I was painted as the foolish, promiscuous girl whose night out went too far and was filled with regret the next day. Or as the girl who couldn't admit to losing her virginity at fifteen, so she made up a story to excuse herself.

I wish I could say I had the strength to try. But I didn't.

Some sexual aggressors amass fifty to sixty victims in their lifetime. If I had reported either of the men who abused me, if I had tried to beat the odds, would other women have been spared?

How am I to forgive myself for that?

In Leslie Jamison's 2014 essay 'The Grand Unified Theory of Female Pain', she wrote:

> I think dismissing female pain as overly familiar or somehow out-of-date – twice-told, thrice-told, 1001-nights-told – masks deeper accusations: that suffering women are playing victim, going weak, or choosing self-indulgence over bravery. I think dismissing wounds offers a convenient excuse: no need to struggle with the listening or telling anymore.

It's that simple. The notion that women are not to be trusted is the balm we use to excuse us from struggling with the listening or the telling. We can't afford to let it go. To open the floodgates. How, then, would we live with ourselves?

A 2011 study by Ohio University found that 66 per cent of respondents agreed with some combination of what the literature calls 'rape myths', including that women lie about rape, that women secretly desire rape and that victims ought to be blamed for their sexual assaults. Bear in mind that this 66 per cent are only the respondents who were willing to acknowledge explicitly their attachment to these beliefs.

We accept these myths in order to excuse ourselves from the burden of meaningfully engaging with the truth of abuse, the inconvenient fact of women's suffering.

A 2007 study by the Australian Institute of Criminology found that one quarter of participants believe that false claims of rape are common. These participants may go on to become jurors in rape cases, and the same study also showed that jurors in sexual assault cases, unlike other types of crime, are likely to bring their own beliefs and attitudes about rape to bear on their deliberations.

On the other hand, we frequently hear about successful convictions for sexual homicide offenders – that is, perpetrators who both rape and kill their victims. This sheds a truly grotesque new light on B.B. King's famous lines: 'Don't ever trust a woman / Until she's dead and buried.'

The idea that women lie about rape also contributes to it being criminally under-reported in every jurisdiction. It is why the majority of sexual assaults go unreported for years, or decades. Some stories of assault are never told to anyone. They are forever unspeakable. They go to the grave with their victim.

How many truths have we lost to the myth of the duplicitous woman? How many stories of abuse are forever silenced when they are buried with the bodies of the girls and women for whom the indignity was unliveable?

In Bri Lee's book about the legal treatment of sexual assault complainants, *Eggshell Skull*, she reflects on the warnings judges are obliged to give juries in relation to certain crimes. One of them is 'Bear in mind this warning: the mere fact that the defendant tells a lie is not in itself evidence of guilt.' I'd love to know how frequently jurors apply this sentiment to sexual assault complainants, for whom the slightest discrepancy in the recollection of detail is so often taken as proof of her assailant's innocence, as confirmation that she is lying, that the whole story is nothing but a cruel invention.

On this point, Lee suggests that there should be a special warning for sexual assault cases:

Bear in mind this warning: there is a strong statistical probability that you will presume this woman is a liar.

In 2015, the *New York Times* reported four cases in which women made rape allegations and were prosecuted and, in some of these cases, fined and put on probation, for making false rape complaints. Years later, evidence surfaced confirming the men's guilt in each case. Each of the rapes had in fact occurred. But that didn't matter. The truth could not eclipse the fiction.

The 2011 Ohio University study also found that men's belief in these rape myths is itself a predictor of sexually aggressive behaviour. When I say these myths are dangerous, I am not engaging in terms of abstraction: the attachment to these myths about rape directly correlates with increased prevalence of rape itself. So the myth of the woman or child who lies about abuse both silences victims and encourages perpetrators in one fell swoop. A potent poison indeed.

What the story of Larry Nassar tells me, and what the story of my own childhood tells me, and what writing this book has taught me, is this: the compulsion to presume that women and girls lie about abuse is systemic. It creates, and recreates, and reinforces, silence. It is the oxygen of shame. It cares little about the idiosyncrasies of our situation or the individual traits of any one perpetrator or victim. It is a gas that adapts to whichever container it finds itself in. It keeps everything in order. It ensures we do not have to bear the discomfort of the listening or the telling. It is a fatal convenience.

In April Ayers Lawson's essay 'Abuse, Silence and the Light That Virginia Woolf Switched On', she reflects on why we are so committed to believing that abuse is imagined. She writes:

For quite some time, it has felt much safer to many people to attribute abuse to fantasy or the need for attention than to face the possibility that it's real.

I think she's right. It's the desperate need for denial that makes enforced silence so powerful, so complete. It's because the stakes are so high: if we allow ourselves to acknowledge the truth, even a fraction of it, the entire house of cards will fall. We will be forced to see clearly what I now see: that abuse has been accepted for so long that it has become a pathology. That violence is everywhere. That culpability is rampant. That abuse kills. That silence kills. That we as women are so unlikely to survive.

As a result, Lawson writes, the victims become encouraged to swallow the truth, to deny it even to ourselves. Especially to ourselves.

If Lawson has correctly diagnosed the compulsion to make abuse unspeakable, if she is right in suggesting that the thing that keeps it alive is our inability to face the fact of it – which I think she is – then there is only one solution. Face it we must.

And so I must forgive myself. I must release myself from the spectre of the victims I didn't protect. Because now I know I couldn't have kept them safe, even if I tried. If the shame hadn't silenced me, others' disbelief would have done so in its place. Our culture of shaming and disbelieving women is bigger and more powerful than any one of us. Because I lived in that world, there was nothing I could do. I know that now.

Once a fellow gymnast was sitting down on the gym floor next to me, stretching, her legs out in front of her, toes pointed to perfection. But she seemed bemused, as if she was daydreaming. I sat down next to her and asked her what she was thinking about. I just realized my legs only go out to here, she said, touching her toes. I just realized how small I am. I can't believe this is where I begin and end.

I now know, all these years later, that during this time in her life she was being abused by the same man who was abusing me.

I thought at the time these were the internal musings of an athlete who spent so much time thinking about her body and its functionality. But now I wonder if I had in fact intruded on a profound moment of her own loss of proprioception: whether her abuse had caused her physical form to disintegrate, to become disembodied, right there in front of me.

VII

Acceptance is a small, quiet room.

Cheryl Strayed, *Tiny Beautiful Things*

REFLECTIONS

As I write this, my tremors have returned and I am terrified that someone might notice. Sometimes I have to take breaks because my fingers won't hit the right keys. The pain is still debilitating at times. Some days I still brush my teeth with blood. Like trauma itself, the process is cyclical and uncertain, lacking clear boundaries, clear finish lines.

There are some days I still want to die; some days I still wonder if there is something cold and rotten inside me that will condemn me to a life of cruelty. There are some days when my Crohn's disease is so bad I can't get out of bed, and I get so lonely, and so angry at how little people try to understand, and I feel like giving up.

On those days, I think about the concluding words

of Bri Lee's memoir about her own disclosure of sexual abuse:

> What do you do in the months and years that follow? When winning the battle has only opened your eyes to the breadth of the war? You cry and you cry, and when you're done crying, you wipe your eyes, and slap your cheeks, and you get angry, and you get to work.

So this book does not necessarily have a happy ending. But it does have a hopeful one: I know I am capable of wiping my eyes and slapping my cheeks, and getting angry, and getting to work.

Here's what I've learned from that work. Violence is a systemic disorder that ruins life after life after life. It is pathological. It is as ubiquitous as it is veiled. This is not just a failure of any single predator. It is a failure of the grandest scale. But more pathological still is our compulsion to ignore it, to erase it, to make it invisible. The truth is that silence is the darkest of captivities. It is ruinous and gratuitous and wretched.

So what do you do, when you discover how much culpability there is, just how many layers this disappointment has?

What do you do when winning the battle has only opened your eyes to the breadth of the war?

There are so many structural problems facing victims

of violence and many of them will take years, decades, generations, to fix. Failures of the law and the justice system, of education, of the healthcare system, of the government, of our culture. I do not have any of these answers. I don't know where to begin.

But I have a head start: I am lucky that in some ways what happened to me was a blinding anomaly, a random act of violence committed by a stranger in the night. Statistically, most acts of sexual violence are not isolated; they are visited upon us by people we know and trust, in circumstances where social and interpersonal dynamics may complicate a survivor's understanding of their trauma, or the boundaries of consent may feel harder to determine clearly.

I have the incalculable fortune of being born into a body that I wanted; the one that aligns with my gender identity and feels as though it fits me the way it's supposed to. I was born middle class and white and the impact that has had on my ability to get help, to be taken seriously, to recover, cannot be underestimated.

If just one of these factors had not aligned in my favour, I might not have been able to get better. I would not have been able to choose Elena. I might, by now, have been dead and buried. Because I am so fortunate in these ways – because I am still alive – it is my duty to testify. To prove that x does not always equal x.

It is harder to be seen than it is to be invisible. It is harder to bear witness to suffering than it is to analyse it. Until we are ready to do that, change will evade us.

As Sally Rooney's protagonist tells the reader in the closing moments of *Conversations with Friends*: You have to live through things before you understand them. You can't always take the analytical position.

A few years ago, Peter Levine was on his way to a friend's sixtieth birthday party. It was a clear winter's day in southern California. As he stood on the side of the road, he was hit at high speed by a teenage driver. He held his breath and waited for help. Somehow, he was wrenched out of the rubble and into an ambulance. The paramedics tried to sedate him.

No, he whispered firmly.

He lay on the stretcher and felt his body shake uncontrollably, as if from the inside out. His mind replayed the moments before the accident, again and again, as if it were still happening. He watched this like a videotape and he let it consume him. He let his legs and arms swing violently until the panic started to fade. Until his muscles finally registered that it was over.

After some moments, his body became still again.

Peter Levine has been a psychiatrist his entire career and has specialized in trauma studies for thirty years. Because of his own trauma research he knew that if he stayed conscious, he could treat his trauma symptoms immediately. While there was still time. He knew exactly what to do to discharge all the fight-or-flight energy that had built up in his muscles in those moments. He let himself relive it, let his body lurch, again and again until the panic left him.

He allowed himself to sit in fight-or-flight mode for as long as he needed, and then it was over. Levine did not develop any symptoms of post-traumatic stress disorder as a result of the accident.

Levine's groundbreaking research about healing trauma has been used in hospitals across the world. Thanks to him, it is now widely understood that if the first moments, or perhaps hours, after a traumatic event are managed properly, it's possible to prevent the majority of long-term symptoms.

What Levine figured out was that if you allowed yourself to be scared, to process the memory in its immediate aftermath, to let the body hurt until it doesn't hurt any more, the memory no longer stays alive inside you.

In 1965, a young man named Tom graduated from high school and joined the US armed forces. He thrived in basic training and looked forward to a career as a lieutenant.

In 1968, Tom was deployed to Vietnam. He witnessed a group of his close friends die. When he returned home, he pretended to live a normal life but soon became plagued by nightmares. He would replay the moments preceding their death again, and again, and again.

If he abandons them – if he stops having the nightmares – then his friends will have died in vain, Tom told Bessel van der Kolk, the psychiatrist who wrote *The Body Keeps the Score*. He couldn't let the memory go because he thought staying in that moment would keep his friends alive.

Ten years later, he barely recognized himself. He began having to sequester himself from Fourth of July holidays because the sound of fireworks would send him into a rage that he could not control. Whenever this part of him was triggered, he became uncontrollably angry. He became violent. He began hurting his wife and two children.

That's when he found Dr van der Kolk. After just six months of highly specialized trauma therapy, Tom's rages vanished. So did the nightmares. He says that since he finished his treatment, he has never felt afraid that he might hurt his children.

It is a cold night but I am on fire. I am shaking so much I feel as though my physical form is dissolving. My friends rush to my side and hold me. I do not try to catch the sobs in my throat. I howl.

I breathe the only words I can muster: He hurt me.

Instead of rolling my dress between my legs, I let myself bleed on the pavement. When I try to stand up

I clutch my ribcage in agony and stumble. I hold on to my chest as if it might snap, I feel the bruises and tears, the ripped muscle, the broken bones.

I don't know what to do next so I say it again: He hurt me.

I let my friends climb into the taxi with me and direct the driver to my tree-lined Sydney street. I am still screaming but I am only faintly aware of it.

When we arrive my friends on either side of me help me out of the cab. They take one arm each and help me hobble to the door.

We ring the bell and I hear my parents' footsteps from the living room down the hall. I hear the hum of the ten o'clock news.

By the time they reach the door, I am bent over double, sobbing, unable to catch my breath.

What happened? my mother says.

A man attacked her, my friend replies.

Call an ambulance, she says over her shoulder, and my father picks up the phone and begins to dial.

I am distracted by my reflection in the glass window when a man walks up and asks me my name.

Lucia, I say quietly, still distracted.

He steps closer to me and I know I should run. He takes my hand in his and pulls me closer.

I do not freeze when he touches me. I do not slip into my practised state of disembodiment and wait for it to be over. I do not become limp and compliant. I do not stare into space as he leads me away. I do not steel myself against his touch.

I rip my hand from his and I run.

I am the frog who jumps straight back out.

The taxi is dark and smells like vomit and the road ahead of me is spinning. I am digging my nails into my stomach so hard that I break the skin. I bite my bottom lip to stop my cries from escaping. I draw blood.

The driver does not ask me for an explanation and I do not offer one. We drive in silence. His organic, mine manufactured from tight jaws and fingers like daggers and a bloody tongue.

He pulls up in front of my house. I live on a quiet street and there is no one around. My bedroom is right at the back of the house, like an extension. I have my own bathroom. I also have my own side entrance that allows me to slip into my room unnoticed.

I limp down the side path and duck when I reach the living-room window, so my parents do not catch a glimpse of me behind the ten o'clock news.

I can feel that I am bleeding down my legs and I pray that none of it reaches the pavement. The last thing I need is a trail, drops of blood leading back to the gingerbread house.

I turn the key in the side door and push it silently. The TV is loud and my parents don't sense my arrival. I duck into my bedroom and stand there for a moment, just staring. I suddenly become aware of the blood again and I limp into my bathroom and lock the door.

I turn on the shower and wait for it to run hot. I try to stand underneath the jets but I am too weak. I let my back fall against the tiles and I slide onto the floor, blood pooling around my Dove soap bar and collecting near my upended bottle of conditioner. I don't know what to do with my hands.

I let the water wash over me for many long minutes. A cracked tile catches my eye and I think about the dull sound that thick glass makes when it smashes.

I make the shower hotter and hotter until it numbs me. I stand up sheepishly and wrap myself in a towel. With the towel still around me, I crawl into bed and lay completely still. I wake up cold and damp, wrapped in a towel and, on top of it, a duvet. I feel disoriented. I smell cigarette smoke and immediately jump back into the shower to wash my hair.

I have to make sure no one can smell it on me.

The difference between me and the accident victim, me and the veteran, is one of kind, not of degree. Their trauma was addressed, not because it was more harmful than mine, but because those men had access to words to lock their experience inside of; words they weren't afraid to say out loud. Words that landed softly on the ear, that did not invite discomfort or disgust; words that ushered in unbridled sympathy.

Words like 'car' and 'accident'. 'Gunfire'. 'Veteran'. Words like 'call an ambulance'.

These men's experiences had a language, a dialect. Mine was unspeakable.

There are so many predators in the world, but silence itself may be chief among them. It is deadly. When it comes to recovery, silence is the knife edge between illness and health. Between dignity and indignity. For some, between life and death.

I cannot eradicate violence. I cannot protect all women and girls from its ubiquity. I cannot even protect myself. No one can. Violence is indiscriminate. It is impervious to vigilance and contingency plans. It does not care that you took the long way home to stay closer to the high street.

Violence lives outside its victims. It is endemic and self-sustaining and probably permanent. I wish I could cure us of it, but I can't.

Because the truth is that if I had stayed home that night in 2007, it is more likely than not that something like this would have happened in another time and place. If I had stayed home that night, it is more likely than not that the man with the knife would have assaulted someone else. Changing our behaviour will never change the fact of violence. As victims, we cannot eliminate violence because we did not create it. It existed long before us, and will continue to exist long after.

There is nothing I could have changed about myself or my life to stop this from happening to me. That is the one thing I finally know to be true.

But there is one thing we can change: the words we wrap it inside of. The words we use to fill the silence.

I have spent ten years wishing I could disappear. I have tried every way imaginable to erase my life, to outrun myself, to make a sacrifice out of myself, always searching for the most profound and permanent act of disappearance. But I cannot, and I will not. Because to be invisible is to give up the only tangible thing I have to offer: this cautionary tale.

I'm a writer. I can't change the world. What I can change is the size of silence. The weight of it. The way it pulls us under.

Trying to erase this experience was the surest way to let it define me. I wish I had known that. But I didn't, and so I said nothing. When I did find a way to tell the truth, it was too late. My intervention was impotent against a body frozen with fear and decayed by disease. Full recovery will never be possible for me because no one, least of all me, wanted to struggle with the listening or the telling. Because no one, least of all me, wanted to face the possibility that it was real. Because of my silence the damage done to me is irreversible. The truth of my life was expressed best by Chelsea Williams during the trial of Larry Nassar: *There will never be a time when I am not recovering.*

This is not the story I would have chosen. It's not the story I would choose for anyone. But it's the one I've got, and it's too late to rewrite it, and I've found a way to live with that. All I can do is tell it, and hope that being honest about what I've lost might help women and girls speak up while recovery is still possible for them.

Acceptance is a small, quiet room.

BIBLIOGRAPHY

Armstrong, Ken and Miller, T. Christian, 'When Sexual Assault Victims Are Charged With Lying', *New York Times*, https://www.nytimes.com/2017/11/24/opinion/sunday/sexual-assault-victims-lying.html.

Atkinson, Meera, *Traumata*. Brisbane: University of Queensland Press, 2018.

Atwood, Margaret, *The Handmaid's Tale*. New York: Anchor Books, 1998.

Ayers Lawson, April, 'Abuse, Silence, and the Light That Virginia Woolf Switched On', London: *Granta* Magazine, 2018.

Backman, Ann-Sofie; Blomqvist, Paul; Lagerlund, Magdalena; Carlsson-Holm, Eva and Adami, Johanna, 'Characteristics of non-urgent patients', *Scandinavian Journal of Primary Health Care*, 26:3, pp. 181–87, 2008.

Baird, Blythe, 'For The Rapists Who Called Themselves Feminist', Button Poetry/YouTube, 2018, https://www.youtube.com/watch?v=LJRKJ_z9iAk.

Bolin, Alice, *Dead Girls: Essays on Surviving an American Obsession*. New York: HarperCollins, 2018.

Borysenko, Joan, *Minding the Body, Mending the Mind*. Carlsbad, California: Hay House, 2005.

Brown, Brené, *Daring Greatly: How the Courage to Be Vulnerable Transforms the Way We Live, Love, Parent, and Lead*. New York: Gotham, 2012.

Brown, Brené, *Listening To Shame*. TED/YouTube, 2012, https://www.youtube.com/watch?v=psN1DORYYV0.

Butler, Octavia E., *Parable of the Talents*. New York: Warner Books, 2001.

Chen, Esther H.; Shofer, Frances S.; Dean, Anthony J.; Hollander, Judd E.; Baxt, William G.; Robey, Jennifer L.; Sease, Keara L.; Mills, Angela M., 'Gender Disparity in Analgesic Treatment of Emergency Department Patients with Acute Abdominal Pain', *Academic Emergency Medicine*, 15:5 pp.414–18, Wiley, 2008, doi:10.1111/j.1553-2712.2008.00100.x.

Coulter, Kristi, *Nothing Good Can Come From This*. New York: FSG Originals, 2018.

Day, Elizabeth, *How To Fail: Everything I've Ever Learned From Things Going Wrong*. London: Fourth Estate Books, 2019.

Dick, Kirby and Ziering, Amy, *The Hunting Ground: The Inside Story of Sexual Assault on American College Campuses*. New York: Hot Books, 2016.

Edwards, Katie M.; Turchik, Jessica A.; Dardis, Christina M.; Reynolds, Nicole; Gidycz, Christine A., 'Rape Myths: History, Individual and Institutional-Level Presence, and Implications For Change". *Sex Roles*, 65:11–12, pp. 761–773, . Springer Science And Business Media LLC, 2011, doi:10.1007/s11199-011-9943-2.

Falley, Megan, 'Holy Thank You For Not', YouTube, 2017, https://www.youtube.com/watch?v=UFo1_KAoM0w.

Fenton, Siobhan, 'How Sexist Stereotypes Mean Doctors Ignore Women's Pain', *Independent*, https://www.independent.co.uk/lifestyle/health-and-families/health-news/how-sexist-stereotypes-mean-doctors-ignore-womens-pain-a7157931.html.

Ferrante, Elena, *My Brilliant Friend*. New York: Europa Editions, 2012.

Ferrante, Elena, *The Story of a New Name*. New York: Europa Editions, 2013.

Ferrante, Elena, *Those Who Leave and Those Who Stay*. New York: Europa Editions, 2014.

Ferrante, Elena, *The Story of the Lost Child*. New York: Europa Editions, 2015.

Foster Wallace, David, *Infinite Jest*. London, Abacus, 1997.

Gay, Roxane, *Hunger: A Memoir of (My) Body*. London, HarperCollins, 2017.

Gouk, Anna, 'Only One Rape in Every 14 Reported in England and Wales Ends with Conviction', *Mirror*, https://www.mirror.co.uk/news/uk-news/only-one-rape-every-14-11323783.

Healthline (contributor), 'Is There a Gender Bias Against Female Pain Patients?', *Huffington Post*, https://www.huffpost.com/entry/is-there-a-gender-bias-against-female-pain-patients_b_589b6b3ee4b061551b3e06ab.

Herman, Judith, *Trauma and Recovery: The Aftermath of Violence – From Domestic Abuse to Political Terror*. New York: Basic Books, 2015.

Hoffman, Diane E., and Tarzian, Anita J., 'The Girl Who Cried Pain: A Bias Against Women in the Treatment of Pain', *Journal of Law, Medicine & Ethics*, 29, pp. 13–27, 2001.

Hunt, Kate; Ford, Graeme; Harkins, Leigh and Wyke, Sally, 'Are Women More Ready to Consult Than Men? Gender Differences in Family Practitioner Consultation for Common Chronic Conditions', *Journal of Health Services and Research Policy*, 4:2, pp. 96–100, SAGE Publications, 1999, doi:10.1177/135581969900400207.

Jamison, Leslie, *The Empathy Exams*. London: Granta Books, 2015.

Jamison, Leslie, *The Recovering: Intoxication and Its Aftermath*. New York: Little, Brown and Company, 2018.

Kaur, Rupi, *Milk and Honey*, New Jersey, Andrews McMeel Publishing, 2015.

Kaur, Rupi, *The Sun and Her Flowers*. London: Simon & Schuster UK, 2017.

Khakpour, Porochista, *Sick: A Memoir*. Edinburgh: Canongate Books, 2018.

Krasnostein, Sarah, *The Trauma Cleaner: One Woman's Extraordinary Life in Death, Decay and Disaster*. Melbourne: Text Publishing, 2018.

Lee, Bri, *Eggshell Skull*. Sydney, Australia: Allen & Unwin, 2018.

Levine, Peter, *In an Unspoken Voice: How the Body Releases Trauma and Restores Goodness*. Berkeley, California: North Atlantic Books, 2010.

Levine, Peter, *Sexual Healing: Transforming the Sacred Wound*. Louisville, Colorado: Sounds True Publishing, 2003.

Levine, Peter, *Trauma and Memory: Brain and Body in a Search for the Living Past – A Practical Guide for Understanding and Working with Traumatic Memory*. Berkeley, California: North Atlantic Books, 2015.

Levine, Peter, *Waking the Tiger: Healing Trauma*. Old Saybrook, Connecticut: Tantor Media, 2016.

Lifton, Robert J., *History and Human Survival*. New York: Random House, 1970.

Lutz, Tom, 'Victim Impact Statements Against Larry Nassar: "I thought I was going to die"', *Guardian*, 24 January 2018, https://www.theguardian.com/sport/2018/jan/24/victim-impact-statements-against-larry-nassar-i-thought-i-was-going-to-die.

Mailhot, Terese Marie, *Heart Berries: A Memoir*. Berkeley, California: Counterpoint, 2018.

Maté, Gabor, *When the Body Says No: The Cost of Hidden Stress*. London: Vermillion, 2019.

Nelson, Maggie, *The Argonauts*. Minneapolis: Graywolf Press, 2015.

Nelson, Maggie, *The Red Parts: A Memoir*. Minneapolis: Graywolf Press, 2016.

Rogers, Annie, *The Unsayable: The Hidden Language of Trauma*. New York: Ballantine Books, 2007.

Rooney, Sally, *Conversations With Friends*. London: Faber & Faber, 2017.

Smith, Zadie, *Swing Time*. London: Hamish Hamilton, 2016.

Strayed, Cheryl, *Tiny Beautiful Things: Advice on Love and Life from Dear Sugar*. London: Vintage, 2012.

Taylor, Natalie, *Juror Attitudes and Biases in Sexual Assault Cases*. Canberra: Australian Institute of Criminology, 2007.

van der Kolk, Bessel, *The Body Keeps the Score: Brain, Mind and Body in the Transformation of Trauma*. London: Penguin Random House, 2015.

Wolynn, Mark, *It Didn't Start With You: How Inherited Family Trauma Shapes Who We Are and How to End the Cycle*. New York: Viking, 2016.

Yanagihara, Hanya, *A Little Life*. New York: Doubleday, 2015.

ACKNOWLEDGEMENTS

Writing this book was the most difficult thing I have ever done, and any words of thanks to those who supported me through it will seem inadequate. But I will try my best: Thank you to Ellah Wakatama Allfrey, for taking a chance on me, and to Ellah, Susie Nicklin, Alexander Spears and the rest of the team at Indigo for supporting me through this process, keeping me going and making me a much better writer. Your help, support and guidance changed my life in so many ways. My gratitude is endless. Words fail.

Thank you to my family, without whom I could never have chosen Elena. I couldn't have done any of this without the support network I have, without the family members I also get to call my best friends, and that fact will forever humble me and make me incredibly grateful.

Thank you to all the dear friends who kept me afloat during this difficult year. To FBC, and everyone who read early drafts of the essay and early drafts of this book. Thank you to those same people, who taught me everything I know about bravery, and who taught me everything I needed in order to start – and finish – writing this book.

Thank you to my doctors, whose support and dedication taught me, again and again, that it is okay to ask for help. That it is okay to ask for more help. This is the lesson I took from this process that will stay with me the longest. So to Kamal, Tanya, Surya and all my other treating doctors and specialists.

Thank you to all the dedicated writers, editors and artists who made the original piece what it was. Very special thanks to Justin and Jini at the *Lifted Brow* for staying up all night with me. Thank you to Hayley Gleeson and Julia Baird at the ABC, and thank you to Amani Haydar for the illustrations that brought the original piece to life. Thank you to Michael Salu, who created the cover artwork for this book. It is an image I will never forget.

And, of course, thank you to Saturn.

ABOUT THE AUTHOR

Lucia Osborne-Crowley is a journalist, essayist, writer and legal researcher. Her news reporting has appeared in ABC News, *Guardian*, *Huffington Post*, *The Wall Street Journal* and *Women's Agenda*. Her long-form writing has appeared in *The Lifted Brow* and *Meanjin*. *I Choose Elena*, based on her celebrated essay in *The Lifted Brow*, is her first book. She lives in London. Lucia's next book, *My Body Keeps Your Secrets*, will be published by The Indigo Press in 2020.

THE

INDIGO

PRESS

Sign up for our newsletter and receive exclusive updates, including extracts, podcasts, event notifications, competitions and more.

www.theindigopress.com/newsletter

Follow The Indigo Press:

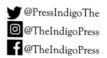

🐦 @PressIndigoThe
📷 @TheIndigoPress
📘 @TheIndigoPress

Subscribe to the Mood Indigo podcast:

www.theindigopress.com/podcast